Hardship and Health in Women's Lives

HILARY GRAHAM

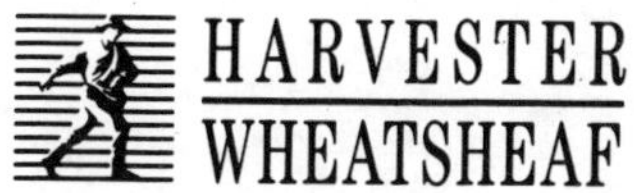

New York London Toronto Sydney Tokyo Singapore

First published 1993 by
Harvester Wheatsheaf
Campus 400, Maylands Avenue
Hemel Hempstead
Hertfordshire, HP2 7EZ
A division of
Simon & Schuster International Group

Typeset in 10/12pt Times and Optima
by Columns Design and Production Services Ltd,
Reading

Printed and bound in Great Britain by
Biddles Ltd, Guildford and King's Lynn

British Library Cataloguing in Publication Data

A catalogue record for this book is available from the British Library

ISBN 0–7450–1264–7 (hbk)
ISBN 0–7450–1265–5 (pbk)

---

1 2 3 4 5 97 96 95 94 93

CONTENTS

FIGURES

TABLES

ACKNOWLEDGEMENTS

I would like to thank the University of Warwick for giving me study leave to start this book and one or two close friends for keeping me going when I began to wonder whether I would finish it.

I am very grateful to those who helped me with different parts of the book: Saul Becker, Nasa Begum, Annie Phizacklea, Nick Spencer and Shantu Watt. I would also like to record my thanks to Sonia Conmy and Karen Prescott who typed and retyped their way through the manuscript.

Thanks are also due to the following for permission to reproduce substantial extracts: the contributing authors of *Alone Together: Voices of single mothers*, edited by Jenny Morris (London: Women's Press, 1992); Taking Liberties Collective, *Learning the Hard Way: Women's oppression in men's education* (London: Macmillan, 1989).

INTRODUCTION

There are around 16 million women in Britain aged 16 to 59. A total of 6 400 000 live in households with children under 16, representing 40 per cent of all women under retirement age (*Employment Gazette*, 1990). Among these 6.4 million women are stepmothers, foster mothers and women living with children within some more informal caring arrangement. The vast majority of women living in households with children, however, are mothers looking after their own offspring.

Hardship and Health in Women's Lives explores the lives of these 6 million women. It is particularly concerned with their domestic lives, and with the responsibilities and routines that structure what they do at home. For most women, what they do at home revolves around caring for children. Their caring responsibilities typically include the welfare of male partners as well; for some it extends to the care of other family members. Caring is associated, too, with a broad range of domestic duties, such as housework, laundry and food preparation.

This cluster of domestic routines shapes the experience of motherhood in ways which seem to transcend differences in women's social position and cultural background. Women who occupy very different class positions share a common domestic position as the person who cares for children and the families they live in. Similarly, White mothers, like Asian and African–Caribbean mothers, find their domestic lives bounded by cultural prescriptions which define them as responsible for childcare and household tasks. Mothers can, and frequently do, challenge these prescriptions. However, while some negotiate more help, few achieve an equal partnership. Most of the 6.4 million women living with children under the age of 16 not only live in households with children, they also labour in them, working to look after the home and the health of those who live there.

In exploring their experiences, the book pays particular attention to mothers whose domestic lives are framed by hardship. The chapters which follow are concerned with the struggle to reunite families separated by immigration laws, with the search for housing and the experience of homelessness. They describe the patterns of paid work and the trends in low income and indebtedness. They look, particularly, at what it means to look after children when money is short; where motherhood is structured around a conflict between caring and economising, between trying to protect individual health and trying to ensure the financial survival of the household.

The book focuses on hardship because of social policies and social trends which are making hardship an increasingly common experience for mothers. The regulations governing immigration from the New Commonwealth and non-European Community countries have become increasingly restrictive in recent decades. The housing market is changing in ways which are pushing more women with children into temporary accommodation, and is turning council housing into a residual housing sector where poor mothers live. The labour market is changing, too, increasing the economic pressures on mothers to work but restricting their job opportunities. Reflecting these trends, families with children are increasingly found among the poorest households in Britain. An increasing number depend on means-tested benefits and on loans and credit for the money they need to survive.

In Britain, the concept of poverty is often used to convey a sense of what it means to be barely surviving. The concept is built around the recognition that people need a minimum of material resources if they are to keep themselves going and protect the health of those in their care. This minimum level of resources can be narrowly defined in terms of providing the basic necessities of food, warmth and shelter. However, although aware that poverty often brings hunger, cold and homelessness with it, most people in Britain take a broader view of what poverty is about. They recognise that social and cultural needs, as well as physical needs, are important components of an individual's welfare. They adopt a relative view of poverty, seeing it in terms of how people live and not just whether they survive. In this relative view, living above the poverty line means being able to take part in activities and experiences that others take for granted.

The focus of the book is on mothers who can take very little for granted. However, it describes their lives in terms of *hardship* rather than through the concept of poverty. This is because of the narrow way in which poverty is often represented. It tends to be seen as a question of money, as a minimum level of income below which health is compromised and survival is threatened. Although shortage of money is often the dominant issue in mothers' lives, they are struggling against other kinds of hardship too. Finding ways to live together as a family in Britain is increasingly difficult for many Asian women. It can also be a struggle to find a home and find the energy to look after those who live there. Indeed, working for pay and sorting out childcare in order to do so can be an additional burden. It can be hard, too, to care for your children on less than you need when your own health is poor. It is this sense of the hard times and hard knocks that go with being a mother that is conveyed in the concept of hardship.

The book begins by reviewing the various sources of information on motherhood, noting how these data sources limit as well as enhance our understanding of women's domestic lives (Chapter 1). Mindful of their shortcomings, the book moves on to explore what can be gleaned from surveys and statistics about the conditions in which mothers live and care for children.

Chapter 2 maps out the routes that women take into motherhood; it looks at the increase in lone motherhood and the impact of labour migration from the New Commonwealth on the family lives of Black and White women. Chapter 3 examines the housing circumstances of families against the backcloth of changes in the housing market affecting the availability of tenured accommodation for those on low incomes.

Chapters 4 and 5 are concerned with the everyday care that mothers provide for their families. These chapters look, in particular, at women's responsibilities for the care of young children and the help that they get (and don't get) from others. Chapter 6 describes the increasing involvement of mothers in paid work, setting the current patterns in the context of wider changes in the labour market.

Chapters 7 and 8 are concerned with money. Chapter 7 reviews the sources of income on which women with children rely for their survival, noting how many families depend on state benefits and how more are turning to various forms of credit for the money they need. Chapter 8 focuses on budgeting on a low income, exploring how mothers work to reconcile their health-keeping and housekeeping responsibilities when money is short.

The final two chapters of the book look more directly at the toll that hardship takes on health. Chapter 9 is concerned with the welfare of mothers. It maps their patterns of health and shows how mothers keep on caring in the face of poor health and deepening hardship. It describes the routines and resources mothers use to keep going and looks, in particular, at the role of cigarette smoking in the lives of White women caring for young children when money is short and housing is poor.

In describing their lives, mothers have offered their own testimony to the health-costs of hardship. However, it is national statistics and not personal accounts that stand as the official record of how hardship and health are linked. Among these statistics, it is those relating to deaths among children that have most commonly been taken as an indicator of the health and living conditions of the population. As a postscript to the book's review of mothers' lives, Chapter 10 maps out the patterns of death among children in Britain.

This synopsis of the chapters will have hopefully conveyed something of the book's focus. It is a focus that illuminates some rather than all aspects of women's domestic lives. For example, the hard times that many women experience around sexuality are noted but not explored. The chapters say relatively little about how abusive relationships, now and in the past, affect how mothers feel about themselves and their children. The hard times they highlight, too, are not ones that involve the loss of children. The book does not describe what it means to face the reception of a child into care or to live through a child dying. It does not record women's experiences of losing the custody of their children to their ex-partner or failing in their struggle to bring their children to Britain. The book points to the web of state services that are involved in these kinds of loss but, again, its coverage is partial. The chapters underline the role of the state in regulating and resourcing the everyday lives of families through its policies on housing and homelessness, immigration and welfare benefits. However, the chapters provide less information on how the health and personal social services help to keep families going and keep them together.

One final point about the contents should be noted. The chapters detail women's experiences. The contribution that men and children make to housework and childcare is explicitly addressed in Chapter 5. For the most part, however, they remain shadowy figures in a landscape marked out in terms of what women do for their families. There are clearly other books to be written about health and hardship in fathers' lives, and about how growing up through hard times affects how children experience, and remember, their childhood.

The aspects of motherhood explored in this book point to the similarities in women's lives. The chapters describe how their lives, at home and in the labour market, are shaped by a common set of domestic responsibilities. The chapters highlight, too, how similarity is crosscut by difference and diversity. While sharing a common position as mothers, mothers are not all the same. Most mothers are non-disabled; for some, motherhood and disability are experienced together. Many mothers are living with men; some are living alone and some live with women. The majority of mothers live in nuclear households while others live in households where two or three generations of women and men live together.

Patterns of diversity are overlaid by patterns of change. Mothers are directly involved in many of the social and economic trends that are reshaping Britain: the increase in lone parenthood, the growth of women's employment, and the increasing vulnerability of families to poverty and reliance on benefits. These social and economic trends have inequality as their common theme. In their different ways, they are serving to widen the differences in life chances and in the living standards of mothers in Britain.

In introducing the book, the section below looks in more detail at the questions of diversity and inequality in mothers' lives. The final part of the introduction discusses the language that women have developed to describe their different experiences of oppression in their everyday lives. It outlines, too, the terms used in the book to capture these divergent experiences.

Diversity among mothers

Diversity is evident in the different routes that women take through motherhood. Around one in seven White mothers are bringing up children as lone mothers. Among African and African–Caribbean mothers the proportion is higher; however, only a relatively small proportion of mothers from other Black minority ethnic groups are lone parents (Haskey, 1991a). The evidence suggests that for many White and Black women lone parenthood is a temporary rather than a permanent status: the average duration of lone motherhood for an unmarried woman, for example, is three years (Ermisch, 1989). The movements into and out of lone motherhood suggest that the increase in the numbers of lone mothers is due less to more women choosing a different, but relatively fixed, domestic arrangement. It is more the result of an increasing number of women building and rebuilding different kinds of family units as they move through motherhood.

Some of those recorded as lone mothers in official statistics are women living in lesbian relationships or those living with female friends and relatives. Such relationships fall outside the definition of cohabitation used in government surveys. Because definitions of cohabitation, like measures of marital status, only pick up on women's domestic relationships with men, sexuality is a dimension of difference that goes unrecorded in most surveys. In the absence of information collected from women, reports tend to extrapolate from the oft-quoted figure that one in ten of the population is lesbian or gay and estimate that one in ten mothers is lesbian. It is a proportion considerably above those reported in surveys where women have been able to record their sexuality and the sex of their partner (Graham, 1986; Sexty, 1990; Graham, 1992a). However, given the risks surrounding the disclosure of a lesbian identity, self-reported data are likely to provide an underestimate of how many mothers are lesbian and how many women are bringing up their children in a lesbian relationship. For many lesbian mothers, not coming out may be a way of safeguarding the custody of their children and protecting them against harassment within their schools and communities (Rights of Women Lesbian Custody Group, 1986; Levy, 1989).

> I'm in a lesbian relationship with a woman; I'm very hesitant to describe myself as lesbian because of what that means everywhere else . . . Certainly in terms of Dan it worries me because I know it can be used against me, the fact that I'm already kind of labelled in the sense that I'm unmarried, he is illegitimate; schools pick up on all that kind of stuff despite whether it is a happy home life or not.[1]

Like sexuality, disability is a little-recognised and little-explored dimension of difference among mothers. It is a dimension of difference which, again, embraces a wide diversity of experience. Some women have conditions which affect their mobility; some have sensory impairments; for some, their mental health makes it hard for them to live their lives as other mothers do. Many disabled women have more than one disability (Martin *et al.*, 1988). Some women become disabled in adulthood whereas other women have always been aware that they live in a body that works in different ways to the bodies of most women. Not all disabilities are visible or made public. Women with progressive diseases, including those who are HIV positive, may work hard to keep their condition hidden from all but the trusted few (O'Sullivan and Thomson, 1992).

> I had never met anyone with my disability who was a parent, and for the first few years of my adult life I completely internalised the idea that I wouldn't have a child if that child might inherit my condition. It was only after I had done a great deal of work on my own self-esteem and self-confidence that I realised that this was a complete denial of my own life-experience.
>
> I believe that many disabled people are not as fortunate as I have been in finding enough support to reach this point. Even now, after seven years of being a parent, I sometimes feel as though I snatched something that didn't belong to me, claimed a prize I had not won, and one day soon it would get snatched back and things would be as they should be.[2]

The evidence suggests that women who have been disabled or have had chronic illnesses from childhood are less likely to have children (Wadsworth, 1991). However, more women are challenging the assumption that being disabled means receiving care and not giving it – being a daughter but never a mother. In addition to women who are disabled before they become mothers there are those who become disabled after becoming mothers. In

Morris' survey of women with spinal injuries, over 40 per cent had children at the time of their injury (Morris, 1989). Recent national surveys of disability among women and men found that one in ten disabled people were parents with dependent children. Most of these parents were in their thirties: in this age group, 60 per cent had dependent children (Martin and White, 1988).

Mothers differ not only with respect to their own experiences of disability but also in their experiences of caring for a child with a disability. Like the estimates of disability among adults, national statistics on the incidence of disability among children are based on definitions of disability rejected by many of those in the disability movements (see Chapter 1). The recent surveys of disability suggest that three in every hundred children have a disability; a total of 360,000 children in Britain (Bone and Meltzer, 1989). These estimates refer only to children under 16. Yet, like mothers caring for non-disabled children, mothers with disabled children can find chronological age an unreliable guide to their children's capacity for independence. Instead of a sixteenth birthday marking the threshold of independent living, mothers may find themselves with continuing financial responsibilities. They can also be more heavily involved in the care of disabled children as they get older and it becomes more difficult to involve other relatives (see Chapter 5).

> Having Maresa has made the issue of disability central in my life. I identify myself much more as a parent of a child with a disability than as a single parent. I get a lot of my support in the way of talking things over when I feel confused, or sharing things I feel excited about, from other parents of children with disabilities. It is they who know what I'm talking about, even if their children have different disabilities from Maresa's.[3]

Woven into their experiences of disability are other aspects of women's identity. Mothers differ with respect to their cultural and religious background, and their exposure to and protection from racism. In societies like Britain, the oppression of racism is hard to avoid. It is an oppression which Black mothers work against as they strive to build a social environment that supports and affirms their child's identity. Yet, women's experiences of racism can lie untapped in the traditional measures of 'race'. Rather than self-defined identities like Black and African–

Caribbean, official statistics and government surveys place women in categories defined by the data gatherers (see Chapter 1). While these categories are contested, official statistics and surveys provide the only source of national data. They suggest that 95 per cent of the population identify themselves as White (Office of Population Censuses and Surveys, 1991a). This suggests that one in twenty women (5 per cent) belongs to a Black minority ethnic group, a broad and diverse category which includes Asian and African–Caribbean women together with women of African, Chinese and Arab descent. It also includes women who define themselves as of 'mixed origin' when asked by researchers to record their ethnic identity.

> We are aware of the many problems that we face every day in this society – racism, isolation, discrimination have become part of our daily life and that is a valid reason to fight against it as women. For instance while I was in my country I never thought in terms of the colour of skin. . . . I have found out that here I am Black and it has made me proud of being Black. Did I consider myself Black because the majority of people here are white and I am 'brown'? – No; I never thought about it, what happened was this society with all its racism has made me aware that I am a 'Black foreigner', therefore unwanted, therefore discriminated against. And when I talk about discrimination I mean it. I have never been able to get a job for which I have applied, except for cleaning offices, or as a kitchen porter, and I have applied for lots of them, including one as a community worker.
>
> Well I am glad about my children, my colour and my principles. . . . They too have suffered from racism and isolation, and many have been the times when I have had to give support to my children because they are isolated at school and have had to suffer insults because they are 'bloody foreigners'. Children can be very cruel to other children, but their racism is the same racism that they see in their parents.[4]

Compared with sexuality, disability and 'race', class is a dimension of social position that has long been on the agenda of social research. However, criticism still surrounds the measures used to place women in the class structure. These measures, based on the current or last occupation of the head of household, suggest that the majority of British households with children under 16 are working class. Over half (54 per cent) of the households with children in Britain are headed by a parent whose present or last occupation was a manual one (Office of Population Censuses and Surveys, 1991a).

National statistics provide a guide to the class composition of families headed by a White, non-disabled parent. However, they obscure the different class profiles found among families where the parents are Black. The limited evidence suggests that mothers living with African–Caribbean men and with men who identify themselves as Pakistani or Bangladeshi are more likely to be bringing up their children in a manual working class household (Duffy and Lincoln, 1990; *Employment Gazette*, 1991). Again, while the evidence is sparse, it indicates that mothers who are disabled, like those with a disabled partner or a disabled child, are more likely to be living in a household identified as manual working class (Baldwin, 1985; Martin and White, 1988; Blaxter, 1990). Being disabled, like the experience of being Black, is also linked to significantly higher rates of unemployment and to a greater reliance on benefits (Martin and White, 1988; *Employment Gazette*, 1991).

Social class provides only a rough guide to the material circumstances in which mothers are bringing up children. More direct evidence comes from government statistics on low-income households and households on benefit. These statistics suggest that, at the end of the 1970s, one in eight (12 per cent) of children were growing up in households with incomes which were less than half the average household income. By the late 1980s, the proportion was one in four (House of Commons, 1991). Social security statistics paint a similar, and similarly grim, picture. In the late 1970s, one million children were living in households on supplementary benefit, the precursor to income support (Piachaud, 1986). By the early 1990s, the figure had doubled. Today, there are over 2 million children in households receiving income support; nearly one in five of all children in Britain (Department of Social Security, 1992a). This sharp rise has occurred at a time when the value of means-tested benefits has fallen relative to earnings (Barr and Coulter, 1990). In other words, the relative poverty of those on benefits has increased at a time when more children and parents have found themselves dependent on the state for their survival.

Increasing hardship has been associated with widening inequalities between families with children. The burden of having a low income has been borne by mothers caring for children as a lone parent and by mothers living in households headed by someone who is disabled or unemployed. Government statistics suggest that around one in ten children with a parent in full-time work live in households with incomes below 50 per cent of average income. Among children cared for by a lone mother, like those in families headed by disabled and unemployed parents, around seven in ten are growing up in households with incomes below this 50 per cent threshold (House of Commons, 1991). Clearly inequality, as well as diversity, are deeply structured into the experience of motherhood in Britain.

The language of diversity

Women have worked to develop a language that speaks to their experiences of diversity and inequality. They have drawn on their involvement both in feminism and in other political movements, like the disability movements and the struggles around racism. Out of these movements have come ways of thinking and talking about oppression which confront stereotypes and shift understandings. For example, the language of disability has involved a shift away from terms which separate and stigmatise ('the handicapped') towards a vocabulary that conveys the sense that disabled people are people and are people who experience disability as an essential part of themselves.

The process of renaming has involved taking words with previously negative connotations, like 'lesbian', to assert a positive collective identity. The word 'Black' has been similarly reclaimed as a way of describing a unity of experience of discrimination among people whose skin colour is not white. It is a name which embodies a political statement, a statement about and against the experience of racism. It is often introduced with a capital letter – Black rather than black – to signify that Black is a political category, forged out of social inequalities and not out of biological differences. In a similar way, references to 'race' carry inverted commas, again to indicate that differences in the position and experiences of Black and White in Britain are socially constructed rather than biologically determined.

> . . . think of how profound it has been in our world to say the word 'Black' in a new way. In order to say 'Black' in a new way, we have to fight off everything else that Black has always meant – all its connotations, all its negative and positive figurations. . . . The whole history of Western imperial thought is condensed in the struggle to dislocate what Black used to mean in order to make it mean something new, in order to say 'Black is Beautiful'.[5]

It is recognised that 'saying words in new ways' is not an unproblematic process. Some women can find themselves outside and between the categories that others seem happy to use. They are disabled and Black, lesbian and working class; multiple identities which bring conflicting allegiances and, for some, an enduring sense of belonging nowhere and always being the odd one out. Commentators have noted, too, how words can become restrictive labels. Politically correct vocabularies can be incorporated into people's understandings in ways which pigeon-hole women, implying that they have one set of experiences deriving from the category to which they have been assigned. Thus, 'disabled mothers' and 'lesbian mothers' are represented as distinct categories, with fixed and homogeneous needs which stem, respectively, from their disability and their sexuality.

The problems with labels underline the importance of keeping language fluid and dynamic, open to the different and changing ways in which women understand their experiences. In describing these experiences, the book draws on terms which are currently used by many of those whose lives they describe. Lesbian is used in preference to gay, a term which has increasingly become male defined (as in 'lesbians and gay men'). However, not all women who have sexual relationships with women identify themselves as lesbian. Some women, too, may embrace a lesbian identity privately but need to be clear about where and with whom it is safe to be 'out' publicly. 'Disabled mothers' is adopted in preference to 'mothers with disabilities'. Adding 'with disabilities' can convey the sense that disability is a separate and optional part of a person's identity. Putting 'disabled' first confirms that people are more likely to experience their disability as integral to who they are and how they live (Oliver, 1990). Like other labels, however, it is not one with which all disabled mothers identify or would want to disclose.

> I haven't told my child my status yet, although she's very up on HIV and AIDS. . . . She did ask me if I were HIV positive but I pretended I haven't heard because that was just too much. My main fear for her is first of all that she would get worried if I got a cold or flu. She's been on her own with me all her life so she's a mixture of amazing independence and dependence on me. We're very, very close and I think I'd like to keep that stress away from her as long as I can. Secondly, and just as important, she and most other children in her situation don't have access to peer support. When my mum had cancer she could talk about it in school and with her friends, many of whom had a granny, friend, aunt or mother who had suffered with cancer. She won't be able to do that with HIV or AIDS until the stigma's removed.
>
> I think it's of growing importance to set up groups for children of parents who are HIV or have AIDS or have died of AIDS. It might be a tiny bit easier to tell her if there were such groups.[6]

Hardship and Health in Women's Lives identifies women who were born in the Indian subcontinent and their descendants born in East Africa and in the United Kingdom as Asian. It identifies as African–Caribbean those who were born in one of the Caribbean islands and their descendants born in the United Kingdom. Black is the term used to refer to Asian and African–Caribbean women and to women of African, Chinese and Arab descent. However, as with the other terms adopted in the book, it should be noted that many women in these groups do not identify themselves as Black. Further, there are women, including Jewish and Irish women, who are recorded as White in government statistics and surveys but who, by virtue of their ethnic origin, culture and religion, experience oppression and discrimination. Reflecting its status as a political and not a biological category, White is also given a capital letter.

One other term requires some comment. In describing their domestic relationships, most mothers (and their children) describe themselves as living in families. It is a term that seems to convey the emotional ties that go with living together, embracing the diverse and changing ways in which women organise their domestic lives. Some mothers, however, distance themselves from the concept of family, regarding their domestic relationships as consciously constructed outside and against the traditionally defined family. This concept of family, as right-wing politicians have been at pains to point out, is a unit consisting of a married couple and their children. Although depicted as *the* family, it is a model of family life which represents only one of a range of domestic arrangements that mothers make for their children. This book therefore avoids references to 'the family'. It does, however, adopt the term 'families' as one used by many mothers to describe the domestic units in which they live and care for children.

While the book seeks to use the currently preferred terms, it relies on data which construct diversity and inequality in very different ways. The patterns outlined in earlier sections of the Introduction, like those examined in more depth in the main chapters of the book, derive from government statistics and social surveys. These data sources use measures of social position rejected by many of those involved in what are sometimes called the new social movements.

This might suggest that mainstream data should be rejected as a resource for understanding mothers' lives. However, these data represent the larger part of what is known about the material and social circumstances in which mothers are caring for children. Government statistics and social surveys are the major sources of information on how circumstances vary across the population and change over time. It is thus these sources which track, however inadequately, patterns of inequality in Britain.

The evidence on hardship and health reviewed in the book is gleaned primarily from mainstream research and government statistics. While the text seeks to adopt the currently preferred language of diversity and oppression, the tables represent women's lives through the categories used in official statistics and social surveys. This is clearly a problematic compromise. Yet it is one that provides a sharp reminder that official sources of information represent women in ways that many reject.

Recognising the problems of building understandings in this way, the book begins by describing both the sources and the shortcomings of the data on mothers' lives. As part of this review, Chapter 1 underlines the importance of personal accounts, where women talk about themselves in their own terms. These personal statements are accorded a privileged place in the book. They are woven between the text and the tables as a separate but linked commentary on how mothers experience their daily lives.

Notes

1. Mother quoted in Gordon (1990), p.102.
2. Mason (1991), p.9.
3. McKeith (1992), p.88.
4. Pelusa in Grewal *et al.* (1988), pp.312–13.
5. Hall (1991), p.11.
6. Pearl in O'Sullivan and Thomson (eds) (1992), pp.150–1.

CHAPTER 1

INFORMATION ON WOMEN'S LIVES

1.1 Introduction

This chapter considers the major sources of information on women's lives:

official statistics
social surveys and
personal records

Official statistics refer to the information collected as people pass through the events and experiences in which the state takes a particular interest. Information is typically recorded by state agencies as a by-product of their involvement in people's lives.

In contrast, social surveys are designed expressly for the purpose of data collection. The ten-yearly census aims to survey everyone; more typically, surveys are based on samples of individuals and households, with the findings from these samples generalised to the wider population.

Personal records are the ones that women make of their own lives, either simply for themselves or for others as well. Unlike official statistics and social surveys, these personal accounts are not filtered through the perspectives and procedures of outsiders.

Official statistics, social surveys and personal records are broad categories that overlap with each other. The dividing line between social surveys and personal records, in particular, is often a blurred one. None the less, the typology helps to illuminate the range of data that can be trawled by those seeking to understand more about the circumstances in which women care for children. The section below briefly reviews these three sources of data. As it indicates, official statistics and social surveys provide what are accepted as the facts about women's domestic lives. Among the facts that they highlight are ones relating to inequality. It is official statistics and surveys which record how social divisions such as class and 'race' take shape in women's experiences of health and family life.

Yet, although an essential resource, these sources of data provide a problematic base on which to build an understanding of women's lives. Firstly, there is often a time-lag of several years between the collection and the publication of official statistics and survey data. Insights into women's circumstances in the 1990s are grounded in information relating to the late 1980s. At a time when patterns are changing slowly, such a time-lag may not be a matter for concern. But the pace of economic and social change through the 1980s and 1990s means that even the most recently published data may well provide only an approximate guide to women's lives today. Secondly, and more importantly, official statistics and social surveys record women's lives in ways which women are increasingly challenging. The methods of data collection can exclude those groups most affected by inequality; at the same time, the measures used to define women's social position (their 'race' and class, for example) can mask dimensions which impact directly on their identities and experiences.

The third and fourth sections of the chapter look, in turn, at the questions of who is included and how their lives are represented in official statistics and surveys. In the process, the sections outline the classification systems used to define women's social class, ethnic identity, marital status and their status as disabled or non-disabled women.

1.2 Sources of information

(*i*) *Official statistics*

The term 'statistics' derives from the German *statistik* or state-istics, a term which underlines the role of the state in the collection of social data (Shaw and Miles, 1979). There are two main mechanisms by which the state collects these data: through vital registration and through the returns made by welfare agencies.

Vital registration includes the recording of births, stillbirths, marriages, divorces and deaths. A task undertaken by the Church in eighteenth-century Britain, vital registration is now a civil and compulsory procedure conducted through the offices of the state (Scott, 1990). The data recorded include sex, place of birth and occupational details. A social class is assigned to children at birth registration on the basis of their father's occupation. However, for babies born to unmarried women, the occupation of the father is normally only recorded if he is present at the registration of the birth. As a result, official statistics provide an incomplete guide to the class background of single mothers and their children (see Chapter 2).

The information collected by welfare agencies relate to the customers of their services. They tend, therefore, to record the absence rather than the presence of well-being. The statistics collected include information on benefit claimants, produced through the operation of the social security system, and on those officially recognised and registered as unemployed. Welfare agencies, too, provide much of the routinely gathered data on health. For example, there are systems for recording visits to the doctor and for the notification of infectious diseases. These systems include the voluntary reporting procedures for people infected by the Human Immunodeficiency Virus (HIV) and for people with Acquired Immunodeficiency Syndrome (AIDS). The process of record-keeping is not initiated unless and until help is sought, with people's conditions represented in categories which reflect professional perspectives and priorities rather than their own.

There are, however, sources of information which are not dependent on the intervention of state agencies. Social surveys represent the most significant of these alternative data sources.

(ii) *Social surveys*

Social surveys cover a broad spectrum of research, including both large-scale national surveys and small-scale local studies. Surveys vary, too, in their methods of data collection. Some studies use methods which encourage women to construct their own agenda and speak in their own terms, whereas others use set questions and fixed-choice answers to collect information in a standardised form from everyone. Within the diversity, two types of survey are particularly important sources of information on the domestic circumstances of families. These are the national surveys, which measure patterns over time, and the one-off studies, which give snapshot pictures of life at particular times and places.

The national surveys include the continuous surveys which collect information on an annual basis from a different sample of individuals in private households. Important examples are the General Household Survey, the Family Expenditure Survey and the Labour Force Survey.

The General Household Survey (GHS) is a multipurpose survey including health and health behaviour among its range of topics (Office of Population Censuses and Surveys, 1991a). It deals only with Britain; the equivalent survey in Northern Ireland is the Continuous Household Survey. These two surveys are the only continuing sources of health information that are not based on general practitioner and hospital records. The GHS relies, instead, 'on people's self-assessments of their health condition'.

While people do the assessing, they do so within boundaries set by the researcher. The survey asks about short-term (acute) illness, which is defined as an illness that has involved cutting down on everyday activities, either at the present time or in the recent past. It also asks about longer term (chronic) health difficulties and about people's assessments of their general health over the previous year (see Chapter 9). The GHS also gives periodic coverage of issues not covered on a regular basis. The 1985 survey, for example, included a set of questions designed to identify people who were involved in helping an older, disabled or sick person. The answers provided the first national data set on the provision of informal care in Britain (Green, 1988).

The Family Expenditure Survey (FES) covers the United Kingdom and focuses on household income from earnings, benefits and investments, as well as household spending on such items as housing, food and fuel (Central Statistical Office, 1991). The FES provides the key source of government data on low income, published as tables of households below average income

(House of Commons, 1991; Department of Social Security, 1992b).

Like the FES, the Labour Force Survey (LFS) is based on private households in the United Kingdom (Office of Population Censuses and Surveys, 1991b). While its name may suggest otherwise, it is an essential resource for those seeking to understand more about women's domestic lives. It is currently the most important source of statistical information on the ethnic composition of Britain, informing analyses of family composition and household structure in Britain's majority and minority ethnic populations (Haskey, 1989a; 1990).

Alongside the continuous surveys are a diverse array of one-off studies. They include some important large-scale national surveys, such as the 1985 Health and Lifestyle Survey (HALS) and the series of government surveys of disability carried out in the mid-1980s (Martin *et al.*, 1988; Bone and Meltzer, 1989; Blaxter, 1990). Most one-off studies, however, are focused around particular localities, networks or identities.

There are, for example, the locally based studies conducted under the aegis of local authorities. These include the surveys funded by local councils and district health authorities which map the health and employment experiences of local communities (Duffy and Lincoln, 1990; City of Liverpool, 1991). The seam of literature on caring and poverty, too, is based largely on studies conducted in particular localities, as is the research concerned with how 'race' affects women's daily lives (Stone, 1983; Warrier, 1988; Bhachu, 1991; Phoenix, 1991). Most of these studies are located in London and the home counties; some, however, are based in other parts of the United Kingdom (for example, Evason, 1980; Bradshaw and Holmes, 1989; Eyles and Donovan, 1990).

Other one-off studies are less closely tied to a geographical area. Instead, they draw on women's networks and shared identities to build their samples. For example, a study of 200 women with spinal injuries relied on the membership lists of the Spinal Injuries Association for its sampling frame (Morris, 1989). In a similar way, a study of step parents made contact with informants through the National Stepfamily Association (Hughes, 1991). Networking through shared identities has provided an important resource for self-surveys. In these surveys, the researchers are also the respondents, designing and conducting the study by and for themselves. One example is *Learning the Hard Way*, a book which welds together the accounts of a group of women who met through an access course. The book records their experiences of education and everyday life (Taking Liberties Collective, 1989).

> On the whole, women like us don't write books. If we do, they don't get published. In this book we've included the writings of 57 women. . . . Some of us are married, a few of us live with the women who are our lovers. All but a few of us have children. Many of us are single parents with nobody very much to help us look after our children. Some of us have lost our children, to adoption agencies, to social services, or to ex-husbands. Some of us have direct experience of sexual abuse, alcoholism, drug abuse, domestic violence and prostitution. We are the women that books get written about.[1]

As the traditions of identity based studies and self-surveys remind us, not all survey data come in the form of tables and statistics. One-off surveys are a rich source of qualitative data, where women describe their lives in their own terms. Their first-hand accounts merge into the third type of information identified at the beginning of the chapter. These are the personal records compiled and collected by women other than for the purposes of research.

(iii) Personal records

'Personal documents' is the term frequently used to describe how people record their lives in a material form: in letters and diaries, pictures and photographs, in books and on tape (Plummer, 1983). But there are also the histories communicated orally, telling it like it is through stories and songs.

> How then to express such a complex journey as ours – continuous and discontinuous, collective and individual? . . . Writing . . . details the things that make us what we are. Since these are numerous, many forms of writing are represented in this

> anthology. Poems, short stories, essays, autobiographical and polemical pieces have been chosen by the contributors to express their experience and views. Writing itself is complex, hard to grasp in some forms, more manageable in others, while different idioms lend themselves more readily to the reflection of different facets of reality. How else could a book such as this be?[2]

These diverse expressions of experience are rarely accorded the same status as government statistics and survey data. This is because data collection in Britain, as elsewhere, is guided by a particular view of what counts as scientific knowledge. It is numerical information derived from large numbers of people and recorded in categories defined by the researcher that is most likely to be accorded the status of scientific knowledge. Personal records rarely measure up to these standards, based, as they are, on individuals recording their lives in their own way. They do not produce the large data sets and the statistically significant findings which are the hallmark of scientific research. But, unlike official statistics and much survey data, personal records are produced outside the gaze of official record keepers and data gatherers. They have an existence which is independent of the activities of outsiders. They thus provide a record of communities where daily life has gone unresearched.

Personal records have played an important part in feminist writing, providing a way of 'learning from the history we live' (Lyman, 1981, p.55). They have resourced, particularly, the histories of groups that have found their lives obscured both within mainstream research and within feminist perspectives. Thus, autobiographical accounts have figured centrally in lesbian histories (McEwen and O'Sullivan, 1988; Hall Carpenter Archives, 1989). They have figured, too, in the work of Black women writers. Here, personal records have tracked changes and diversity among Black women, describing the conflicting commitments and different priorities which shape their lives (Bryan *et al.*, 1985; Grewal *et al.*, 1988).

Within the disability movements, too, women are asserting the importance of recording life as it is lived. Creating a fund of knowledge and a body of artistic work is seen as a first stage in the long process of reclaiming identities constructed and controlled by the non-disabled world (Browne *et al.*, 1985; *Feminist Art News*, 1989). This literature on disability is being extended by personal testimonies that record women's experiences of learning about and living with their HIV-positive status (O'Sullivan and Thomson, 1992).

> Our history is hidden from us, as are role-models to whom we can relate. Because the presentation of our experience is constructed by non-disabled people, most of the recording of the lives of disabled people is done in a way which is deeply alienating to us. . . . Once we have found a language to describe our experience, from our point of view rather than that of the non-disabled society, we can assert the experience of disability in our terms.[3]

Personal testimonies and reflections on experience have figured centrally in the so-called new social movements, which include feminism, the struggles against racism, and the lesbian and disability movements. Personal records provide a way for women to understand themselves and to challenge the perspectives of others. However, records which capture subjective understandings do not provide an unproblematic resource from which to build perspectives on women's lives. There are problems about inclusion and representation, about who speaks on behalf of whom. As a number of contemporary anthologies make clear, Black, lesbian and disabled women do not speak with one voice (Browne *et al.*, 1985; Grewal *et al.*, 1988; Hall Carpenter Archives, 1989). The accumulation of many stories and multiple voices provides only a partial solution: some voices may still come through more strongly than others.

The power to speak loudly may reflect material differences between women. While some women may have ways of recording their lives – in diaries, in notebooks, on word-processors – others may leave no trace. Not speaking out may reflect self-silencing, an intentional failure to leave a record of one's existence. Women whose lives come under the surveillance of state agencies are often all too well aware that 'anything they say may be taken down and used against them' (Glastonbury, 1979, p.174).

Silencing can occur in other ways, too. It can occur through the construction of narratives of oppression, which come to be seen as the authentic experience of the group as a whole. These narratives tend to be ones recounted by those vested with authority within community groups and political movements. Divergent understandings tend, as Ann Snitow puts it, 'to be toned down and tuned out'. She points to 'narrative taboos': the things that cannot be said and the understandings that cannot be challenged (Snitow, 1992, p.33). Such taboos can make it hard to understand, let alone to speak about, oneself in other ways.

Exclusion and representation are clearly important issues for those seeking to build understandings of women's lives from personal accounts. However, the problems are not unique to this source of data. As the next two sections outline, official statistics and survey data are constructed in ways which obscure minority viewpoints and experiences, and which mask dimensions of inequality and oppression that women have sought to make visible.

1.3 Who is included?

Official statistics and social surveys seek to provide a comprehensive picture of the health and circumstances of the population. Yet, the procedures they employ can work against inclusiveness. Exclusion can be the outcome of three different processes. It can come about, firstly, from the criteria that govern entry into official statistics and social surveys, criteria which may debar individuals from inclusion or from which individuals may wish to exclude themselves. It can result, secondly, from the statistical procedures used in sampling and data analysis. Thirdly, exclusion can be the result of the non-recording of data on aspects of identity which structure women's understandings of who they are and how they live. These three processes are outlined in more detail below.

(*i*) *Exclusion from entry*

Official statistics based on the administration of welfare exclude those not in contact with welfare agencies. The statistics are thus likely to underestimate the scale of hardship and ill-health in Britain. For example, social security statistics exclude those on low incomes who, while eligible for financial support, are not claimants. The statistics for families on benefit, outlined in Chapter 7, should be interpreted in the context of a significant non-take-up of means-tested benefits (P. Craig, 1991). While government statistics do not give a breakdown of claimants by ethnic origin, the evidence points to under-claiming among Asian households and non-English speaking people (Brown, 1984; National Association of Citizen Advice Bureaux, 1991).

Changes in the regulations governing eligibility also affect the picture of hardship represented in social security statistics. The restrictions placed on the eligibility of 16- and 17-year-olds for income support, introduced in 1988, removed a large group from the statistics altogether. The effects of eligibility criteria are also reflected in unemployment statistics, which only include those officially registered as unemployed. In 1991, there were 2.2 million people officially registered as unemployed. However, another million would have registered if official definitions of unemployment had not changed. It is estimated that a further 2 million people would have liked regular employment, but were not at that time actively looking for work (Millar, 1991).

It is not only official statistics that set conditions around eligibility. The criteria imposed by social surveys also frequently exclude a significant number of people whose lives are touched by the experience under study. National surveys generally seek their respondents from electoral registers and lists of private households. Those who do not make it onto these records are left out. The excluded populations represent some of the most disadvantaged groups in Britain. They include those in hostels, prisons and hospitals, and those living on the streets. The estimated 12,000 Traveller families in England and Wales are also unlikely to find their way into continuous surveys such as the General Household Survey or into the statistics on low income households (Durward, 1990).

People can actively avoid inclusion in social research. A proportion of those contacted refuse to take part or make incomplete returns. The national continuous surveys usually achieve response rates of between 70 and 90 per cent (Central Statistical Office, 1991; Office of Population Censuses and Surveys, 1991a). While few details are released on who opts out of social surveys, the limited information points to lower response rates among Black than among White people. Wariness can be fuelled by concerns that Black experiences will be drained of their meaning and refashioned in ways that can be used against minority ethnic groups (Booth, 1988; White, 1990).

(*ii*) *Too few to count*

As noted in Section 1.2, the model of research governing the production of data on people's lives is one that places a premium on statistical analysis. As a result, social surveys often rely on large samples, selected in ways which make them representative of the population as a whole.

Such studies might be expected to provide a rich source of insight into the lives of minority groups. They involve large numbers of respondents chosen to reflect the diversity of groups within the community. However, most national surveys say little about minority group experiences. This is because the numbers, even with large samples, are insufficient to enable statistically valid analyses to be conducted. As a result, the experiences of lone mothers and disabled women are often not examined separately. The impact of 'race', too, tends to go unexplored. For example, the Health and Lifestyle Survey was based on a sample of 9000 adults and yet the major published reports on the survey provided no insights into the health experiences of Black and White respondents (Cox, 1987; Blaxter, 1990). The OPCS (Office of Population Censuses and Surveys) surveys of disability were similarly based on large and representative samples. The report on disability among adults provides an estimate of the prevalence of disability among Asian, African–Caribbean and White respondents. However, because of the small numbers of Black respondents, no further analyses are provided (Martin *et al.*, 1988).

Researchers have tackled the problems surrounding the analysis of minority group experiences in two ways. Firstly, data from continuous household surveys, like the Labour Force Survey and the General Household Survey, can be aggregated across a number of years. Such aggregated data provide the basis of estimates of the number and composition of Britain's one-parent families, and the profiles of minority ethnic communities in Britain (Haskey, 1990; 1991a).

As a second strategy, researchers have designed studies that increase the proportion of minority group respondents. This approach was adopted in a comparative study concerned with the experiences of parents with disabled and non-disabled children (Baldwin, 1985). It was also the approach used in the national survey of *Black and White Britain* (Brown, 1984). Complementing these comparative studies are ones that focus only on minority groups, often combining a range of sampling methods to increase the number of respondents. Thus, there are studies concerned with lone mothers and lesbian mothers, and with the common and divergent themes in the lives of Asian and African–Caribbean mothers (Evason, 1980; Hanscombe and Forster, 1981; Stone, 1983; Warrier, 1988).

(*iii*) *No records kept*

Some dimensions of identity and inequality are not routinely included in official statistics and social surveys. For example, data on women's domestic lives are collected in ways which make lesbian relationships invisible in most sources of data. Like sexuality, the experience of disability has gone largely unrecorded in studies of household composition and living standards. However, the 1991 census included, for the first time, a question designed to identify disabled and non-disabled people. From the early 1980s, two government surveys, the Labour Force Survey and the General Household Survey, have included a question on ethnic origin. Both use the same form of question and the same categories of response (discussed in Section 1.4). The 1991 census also included a question on ethnic identity, using a set of categories different from the one used in the LFS and GHS.

More extensive data collection raises the question of whether it is in the interests of minority groups to have their existence and experiences made visible in official statistics and social surveys. This question has been debated particularly in the context of 'race' statistics, although the issues it raises are ones which confront other minority groups. On the one hand, it is recognised that measures of 'race' are needed if the nature of racism and the scale of racial disadvantage are to be explored through sources of data that have been used to highlight other forms of oppression. The proxy measures, based on place of birth and parent's place of birth, used in the 1971 and 1981 censuses, no longer provide an adequate substitute (Booth, 1988). On the other hand, more data on 'race' runs the risk of fuelling a process of *racialisation*; this is a process in which 'race' comes to infuse popular and political understandings of social problems. Thus, for example, 'race' has figured centrally in both official statistics and public debates about law and order (Carr-Hill and Drew, 1988). 'Race' statistics played a powerful role, too, in the 'numbers game' constructed around the issue of immigration in the 1970s and 1980s (Ohri, 1988; Solomos, 1989). As Chapter 2 notes, these decades saw increasingly restrictive immigration legislation being passed by governments.

The issues raised by the collection of information on 'race' turn not only on the question of whether such data should be collected, but how experiences forged out of oppression should be represented in official statistics and social surveys. It is this issue that is explored in the next section.

1.4 How are women's lives represented?

In personal accounts, women represent themselves and their lives in their own way. In official statistics, and in most social surveys, experiences and relationships are represented in frameworks constructed by others. The frameworks are designed to enable the same information to be collected from everyone so that each person can be placed into a predefined category: as single, disabled, White, working class. The standardised procedures for collecting and recording information on these social positions enable official statistics and social surveys to measure differences among women and across time. Yet, while tracking inequality, these sources of data can also mask it. This is because the categories researchers use to measure social divisions can fail to capture how extensively and deeply they are carved into women's lives.

There are three problems with the categories used in government statistics and mainstream research. Firstly, they typically treat social divisions, like social class and 'race', as properties of individuals. They are represented as personal characteristics (things people have) rather than social relations (ways people live). Secondly, the classification of social class and 'race', disability and marital status rest on ideological assumptions about where women belong. Thirdly, the classifications turn complex experiences into ordered categories. Women acquire clear, stable and singular identities. For example, they cannot be simultaneously married and single, or be both working class and middle class. These three problems are reviewed briefly in turn.

(*i*) *Properties of individuals*

Much official and survey data relate to social positions and social relations: they try to capture an individual's position in relation to gender, sexuality, class, 'race' and disability. Yet, these dimensions are typically represented in ways which cut them loose from social divisions. They are treated as individual attributes, features which reside in people rather than in their social environment. For example, definitions of disability used in mainstream research centre around what individuals have not got and what they cannot do. The focus is on individual capabilities, not environmental barriers. Thus, the classification used in the OPCS surveys of disability measured an individual's ability to perform activities rather than the social arrangements which prevent people with impairments participating in the everyday activities that others take for granted (Abberley, 1990; Oliver, 1990).

Social class also tends to be treated as an individual attribute. The attribute that individuals possess is occupation, with classifications built around a finely graded hierarchy of occupations. The occupational hierarchy is then used to place people into broad social class groups.

The major social class schema is the Registrar General's classification of occupations. It is based on a sixfold typology, with three non-manual groups (social class I, II and IIINM) and three manual groups (social class IIIM, IV and V) (Table 1.1).

Table 1.1 The social class of some occupations in the Registrar General's classification of occupation.

Social class		Examples of occupations
I	Professional, etc.	Accountant, clergyman, doctor
II	Intermediate	Teacher, farmer, nurse
IIINM	Skilled non-manual	Secretary, shop assistant, sales representative
IIIM	Skilled manual	Bus driver, electrician, miner (underground), cook
IV	Semi-skilled manual	Agricultural worker, assembly worker, postman
V	Unskilled manual	Laundry worker, office cleaner, labourer

The split between non-manual and manual occupations marks the dividing line between middle and working class occupations. The dividing line, like the classification as a whole, reflects the hierarchies in male occupations, where having a non-manual job generally means more money and more status than having a manual job. However, many of the major female occupations, including clerical and shop work, are both non-manual and low paid. Further, there is less sensitivity to the gradations in women's occupations; women tend to cluster in a small number of social classes (and in IIINM in particular) rather than being spread more evenly across the scale.

'Race', too, tends to be treated as a property of individuals rather than of the societies in which they live. Most typologies do not invite people to record their experiences of racism but to define themselves in terms of physical and cultural attributes. Whereas measures of social class rely on one attribute, 'race' typologies typically combine a complex of dimensions into a single scale. As Table 1.2 records, the scales use categories defined only by colour ('White') alongside ones where colour is not the explicit criterion. The other categories relate, instead, to continent or country of origin/birth. It is these dimensions which are woven into the typology used in the Labour Force and General Household Surveys, a typology which 'has come closest to being the standard question used for self-assessment' (Booth, 1988, p.249). As the discussion below indicates, the scale highlights the way in which normative assumptions guide the coding of people's identities.

(*ii*) *Whose realities?*

The classifications do more than convey a sense that 'race', class and disability are properties of individuals. They convey other messages too. Built into the measures of social position are a set of understandings about who occupies the dominant and subordinate positions in British society. The scales provide an insight into the ideologies which shape women's lives.

Take, for example, the classification of ethnic origin. It relies on one category, 'White', to classify people who are indigenous to the United Kingdom or who are of European origin. It is chosen because it speaks, as Heather Booth puts it, 'to the racism of those identifying with it' (Booth, 1988, p.252). The category 'Black' is one with which many African–Caribbean people identify, especially those who recognise their children as Black or Black British. However, the evidence available at the time the scales were being constructed suggested that many Asian people preferred to be classified according to their country of origin and religion (Booth, 1988, p.252). As a result, a composite scale was constructed that combines colour and place of birth in different ways for the White and Black populations (see Table 1.2).

Ideological assumptions underpin class classifications too. A

Table 1.2 General Household Survey and Labour Force Survey measure of ethnic origin.

Respondents are asked to which of the following groups they consider they, and members of their family, belong:
White
West Indian or Guyanese
African
Indian
Pakistani
Bangladeshi
Chinese
Arab
Mixed origin (specify)
Other (specify)

Source: Derived from OPCS (1991b), pp.24, 49.

central tenet of the Registrar General's classification is that women have a different relationship to the class structure than men. Men earn their class position directly through their occupation. Women's position is mediated through their relationships with men. In most official and survey data, married and cohabiting women are given the class ascribed to their partner; only women living outside such relationships with men are allocated a class position on the basis of their own occupation.

Women's ethnic identities are often ascribed in the same way, through the category into which the head of household has been slotted. The analyses provided in Brown's study of *Black and White Britain* and in the Labour Force Survey use a household ethnic identity based on the head of household, with men ascribed the headship of married couple households (Brown, 1984; Haskey, 1989a).

It is a procedure that assumes homogeneity within households: a common standard of living and a common ethnic identity for all members of the household. Assuming homogeneity, it masks diversity within households. It obscures differences in access to material resources within families, differences which can leave women experiencing hidden poverty amidst household plenty. It obscures, too, the many relationships in which partners do not have a shared ethnic identity. Analyses of the 1984–6 Labour Force Surveys suggest that over a quarter of married and cohabiting African–Caribbean women (and men) aged under 30 had a White partner (Central Statistical Office, 1988). Children born to these couples would be counted within the ethnic group in which their father was placed.

Like 'race' and class classifications, marital status categories rest on assumptions about gender relations. These categories seek to identify women's primary domestic and sexual relationships through a classification that accords a privileged status to marriage. Marriage is the lynchpin of the classification, with positions within and outside marriage ranged around it. Women are recorded as married (a category widened to include cohabiting relationships with men) or as never married (single) women, as separated or divorced women, or as widows (Table 1.3). As these categories suggest, it is women's legal status that drives the classification, not the meanings women give to their personal relationships.

Table 1.3 General Household Survey marital status categories.

Marital status
Married
Cohabiting
Single
Widowed
Divorced
Separated

Source: Derived from OPCS (1991a), p.281.

The attention to legal status means that women's domestic and sexual relationships with women are lost altogether. Cohabitation, potentially a category which could make these relationships visible, is treated as a heterosexual category. As the General Household Survey puts it, 'an informant can only be cohabiting with an unrelated adult of the opposite sex' (Office of Population Censuses and Surveys, 1990a, p.262). Two female friends, two sisters, a couple in a lesbian relationship cannot 'cohabit'. They are classified, instead, according to their place outside marriage (as single, separated, divorced or widowed women).

(iii) *Fixed categories*

The coding systems for social class and 'race' are designed to place individuals into one of a set of mutually exclusive categories. The set is seen to cover the range of possible class and 'race' positions that an individual could occupy. Similarly, measures of marital status are designed to provide a comprehensive and exhaustive classification, with clear boundaries between the different identities.

However, women often experience their lives in ways that do not fit into boxes. For example, their sense of their own ethnicity may be more complex and dynamic than the coding systems allow for. Women presented with identities listed in Table 1.2 may find none for themselves. They may have a definition of self that cuts across the categories or lies beyond them. In such circumstances, they must opt for a category that captures only part of their self-identity or define themselves into the residual 'other' ethnic group.

Women's domestic lives, too, may not conform to the ordered world of the marital status scales. As Joan Chandler puts it, 'there is a broad and varied group of women outside conventional marriage but with some domestic connection to men' (Chandler, 1991, p.2). Thus, women in husband-absent marriages are classed as married, while they may, like lone mothers, take sole responsibility for the home and the children. Conversely, a single woman in a stable visiting heterosexual relationship is categorised by her legal status, although she may share more of herself and her life with her partner than many married women do (Chandler, 1991, p.2).

Measures of disability can similarly violate a woman's sense of self. Categories based on what is missing and what women cannot do put the accent on the negative, making it hard to assert a positive self-identity. They assume, too, an unchanging condition and an unchanging environment. Yet, the experience of disability can vary day by day; it varies, too, according to context.

> At home with my family, with my animals, with my lover, I don't feel they condemn me for this mask. And so for a short while I'm allowed to be me, the real me . . .. I only cease to be the person I know I am when I walk down the street. Then I see the look in your eyes. I see your horror and your revulsion. It's like being cut in half.[4]

1.5 Working with the shortcomings

This chapter has examined the sources of information on women's lives. It has noted that what counts as knowledge about women derives primarily from official statistics and survey data. It is these sources, too, that provide information on how dimensions of oppression and inequality, like class and 'race', are related to their material circumstances and health experiences.

Yet, the recognised sources of knowledge about women have limitations. The limitations turn on the questions of who is included in the data sources, and how their lives and identities are represented. As the chapter has suggested, the procedures which determine 'who' and 'how' tend to exclude and misrepresent the lives of those most affected by disadvantage and discrimination.

Problems of exclusion and misrepresentation raise questions about how official and survey data should be used. They raise questions about how to work with data which provide an essential but problematic base on which to build understandings of women's experiences. As outlined in the Introduction, the book adopts a twofold approach.

Firstly, it highlights the limitations of official and survey data, by addressing them directly. The issues raised in this chapter are underscored in the chapters which follow. The tables typically represent women in official categories while the text seeks to represent women in the terms which recognise the changing language of diversity and oppression. Although something of a compromise, it is a strategy that serves as a reminder that official understandings can be seriously out of line with women's understandings of their social position.

Secondly, the book accords a special place to personal reflections, in which women speak and write about their lives in their own terms. It pays particular attention to sources of data where subjective understandings are not filtered through official understandings. These sources of data include both the open-ended accounts recorded by researchers in qualitatively oriented surveys, and the personal records that women produce when out of the reach of survey researchers and official data gatherers. These personal reflections are interspersed between the text and the tables, providing their own commentary on how women represent themselves and make sense of their lives.

Notes

1. Taking Liberties Collective (1989), p.vii.
2. Grewal *et al.* (1988), p.4.
3. J. Morris (1991), pp.184, 187.
4. T. Leslie quoted in J. Morris (1991), p.25.

CHAPTER 2

SETTLING DOWN

2.1 Introduction

This chapter looks at the process of settling down in the context of the social policies and social trends which have reshaped family life in Britain in recent decades. It is concerned, firstly, with the shift away from legal marriage as the setting in which women become mothers and care for children (Sections 2.2 and 2.3). It looks, secondly, at how the process of labour migration from the New Commonwealth affected the domestic lives of Black women who came to Britain in search of work and to join families (Sections 2.4 and 2.5).

2.2 Pathways into motherhood

Vital registration statistics record how women in the late 1940s, 1950s and 1960s followed a similar route through adult life. Marriage was the destination for the vast majority. Women across the class spectrum could expect to be married by their early twenties and remain married until they died. Early and life-long marriage was associated, too, with early motherhood. The majority of women (around 70 per cent) who were married in the mid-1960s had their first baby within three years of marriage (Kiernan, 1989).

From the late 1960s, women's pathways through adult life began to diverge. Getting married and marrying young were no longer the dominant patterns. Today, 70 per cent of women in their twenties are single and trends suggest that the proportion of women who are married is falling (Cooper, 1991). This shift away from marriage has been associated with an increase in cohabitation: one in four (24 per cent) non-married women in their twenties live with a male partner (Office of Population Censuses and Surveys, 1991a). It has been associated, too, with an increase in divorce and in remarriage. If divorce rates continue at their mid-1980s level, over a third (37 per cent) of marriages are likely to end in divorce (Haskey, 1989b). The majority of those who divorce get married again. Over half (53 per cent) of women who divorce are remarried within 6 years; 60 per cent are remarried within 10 years (Office of Population Censuses and Surveys, 1990a).

> One outing in particular stands out from last year as illustrating our positive experiences of companionship. Four of us, single mothers, had travelled down from London to Horstead Keynes in Sussex with our five children, for a bluebell picnic and ride on the preserved steam railway. . . . It wasn't until a long while after that I realised what a wide variety of experiences we and our children had brought with us that day – gay and straight, divorced and unmarried, different ethnic and social backgrounds – and our children are growing up boys and girls in a society radically different from the one experienced by each of their parents.[1]

Like women's approach to marriage, there is greater heterogeneity in women's pathways into motherhood. The last decade has seen a steady rise in the proportion of women who do not have children. Women who have children are having them later, and more are having them outside marriage (Jones, 1991). In the early 1960s, 5 per cent of births in the United Kingdom were to women who were not married. By 1980, the proportion had more than doubled to 12 per cent of total births. By 1990, it had doubled again, to 28 per cent (Jones, 1991). As this figure suggests, more than one in four children in Britain are born to a single (unmarried) woman.

Women are not only shifting away from marriage as the setting in which to have children, more women are also caring for children outside marriage. At the beginning of the 1970s, there were 500,000 lone mothers, representing 7 per cent of all women with dependent children. Today, there are over a million lone mothers, and their number is increasing by around 50,000 a year (Haskey, 1991a). As Figure 2.1 suggests, they represent 15 per cent of Britain's households with children. The majority of lone mothers in Britain are separated and divorced women (see Section 2.3).

> If you begin to rely on someone being there you also begin to believe you can't manage without them. Despite the evidence that you do for most of the day everyday, week in and week out, month after month. Almost as much as financial dependency it kept me in the marriage – how could I go? I'd never manage the kids on my own. In the event I had to . . .[2]

While the increase in births to single women, like the increase in lone motherhood, points to a shift away from marriage, they represent trends and not universal patterns. The majority of births (over 70 per cent) still take place within marriage. Further, birth registration data record that the majority of babies born outside marriage are born to cohabiting couples. Over half of the babies born to single women are jointly registered by both

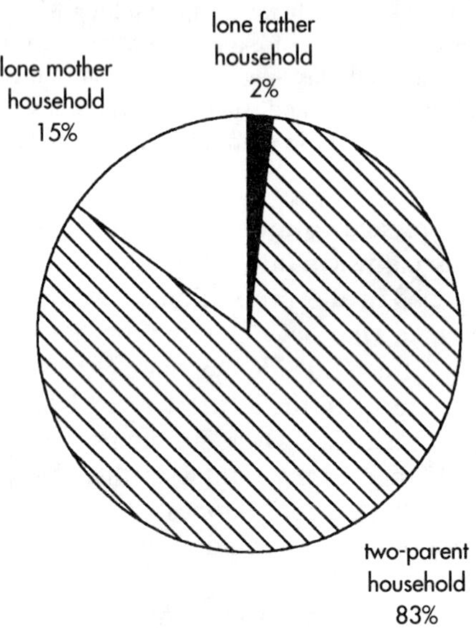

Figure 2.1 Families with dependent children: patterns of one-parent and two-parent households, Britain, 1989.

Note: Dependent children are persons in the family unit who are under 16 or aged 16 to 18 and in full-time education and living in the household.
Source: Office of Population Censuses and Surveys (1991a), derived from Table 2.34.

parents living at the same address (Jones, 1991). Taken alongside the data on births within marriage, this suggests that nearly nine in ten babies are born into households in which their parents are living together, either as a married or cohabiting couple.

The majority (86 per cent) of children in Britain are also brought up in a two-parent and heterosexual household (Haskey, 1991a). In most two-parent households, children are living with their biological parents. However, a growing number of children are growing up in reconstituted (step) families, where their parent's partner is not their biological father or mother. Recent estimates suggest that one in ten children are being brought up in reconstituted families (Kiernan and Wicks, 1990). Building stepfamilies often involves women in negotiating relationships with children who are not their own. The accounts that women have provided of their experiences suggest that being a stepmother can mean setting and achieving particularly high standards of maternal care. Like single mothers, stepmothers find themselves working hard to dent negative stereotypes which cast them as neglectful and uncaring (Hughes, 1991).

> I was a bit wary but I felt quite positive about it (meeting her stepchildren for the first time). I was very nervous, frightened about what they thought of me, not really knowing what my position was, how they saw me, whether they saw me as a threat.

> He would show things to his father he wouldn't show to me. 'You've got your own place why don't you go there'. Slamming back doors shouting 'why don't you sod off'. Of course I used to get upset, very upset, but well, with both of them (husband and stepson) I was determined to care.[3]

Many stepmothers are ex-lone mothers who have moved out of lone motherhood into cohabitation and marriage. The evidence suggests that single mothers are typically on their own for shorter periods of time than separated and divorced mothers. It has been calculated that the mean duration of lone motherhood for single mothers is 3 years; for separated and divorced mothers, it is 5 years (Ermisch, 1989). Reflecting the significant numbers who move on into cohabiting relationships with men, the population of lone mothers contains a high proportion of women who have been caring for children as lone mothers for relatively short periods of time. Analyses of the General Household Survey suggest that 60 per cent of single and divorced women have been lone mothers for less than five years. Among separated women, the proportion is 85 per cent (Haskey, 1991a).

Such statistics point to the enduring significance of marriage as the setting for parenthood. They highlight, too, how diversity is taking shape in mothers' lives. Diversity is partly the result of some mothers setting up long-term domestic arrangements outside marriage. But it is more the result of an increasingly large group of women changing their domestic relationships as they move through adult life. The official sources of data record that, compared with the 1950s and 1960s, more women are experiencing periods of living alone, living with a partner, marrying, divorcing and becoming a lone mother. Individual biographies remind us that the labels ascribed to women ('lone mother', 'married mother', 'stepmother') do not describe a permanent status. They can, instead, represent transitional points in the changing fortunes of women's lives.

> It wasn't until recently when I started to focus on the broader public response to single parents that I realised there were so many hostile criticisms being made of us. My first observation about this response must be that any generalisations about single parents are difficult to make because we are present in so many conditions of society and for some it is just a transitory lifestyle. We have also arrived at the position from so many different directions.[4]

While recognising that generalisations are difficult to make, the section below explores some of the pathways along which women travel into lone motherhood.

2.3 Caring for children alone

The patterns of single and lone parenthood are ones that are deeply gendered. It is women, not men, who have children on their own. It is women, too, who make up the majority of Britain's lone parents. This majority is growing both absolutely and relatively. Not only are there more lone mothers today than there were in the early 1970s, but they make up a larger proportion of the lone-parent population. Nine in ten lone parents in Britain are women (Haskey, 1991a).

As Figure 2.2 suggests, there are two main routes into lone motherhood: having a baby as a single (unmarried) woman and experiencing the breakdown of one's marriage. Around three in ten lone mothers are single women; six in ten are separated and divorced women. Single mothers are the youngest group of lone mothers. The majority were living with their parents before their first pregnancy, moving on, often through temporary accommodation, into local authority housing (see Chapter 3).

Separated and divorced women tend to be older than single mothers, with the majority in their thirties. Most lived previously, not with their parents, but in a nuclear household with their husband and children (Bradshaw and Millar, 1991). Studies suggest, unsurprisingly, that marriages break down because the couple does not get on any more and one or other partner establishes another relationship. For example, in the Bradshaw

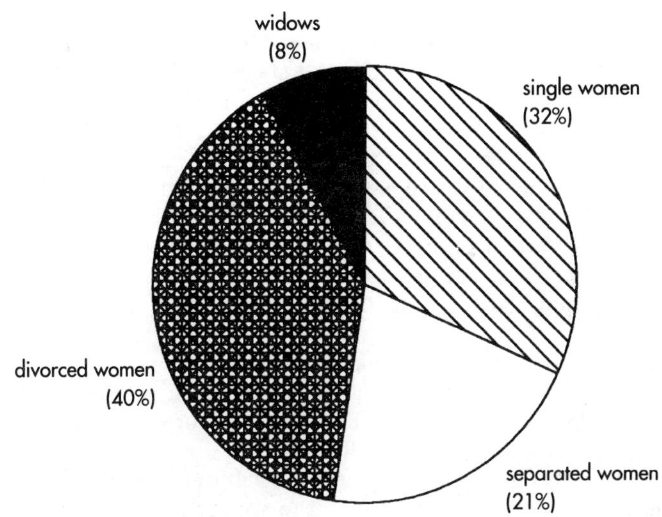

Figure 2.2 Heads of lone mother families with dependent children, Britain, 1987–9 combined.

Note: Dependent children are persons under 16 or 16 to 18 and in full-time education.
Source: Haskey (1991a), derived from Table 2.

and Millar (1991) study of 1400 lone parents, finding another lover or finding that their partner was involved with someone else was the most common reason given for no longer living together. 'Not getting on anymore' was the second most common reason.

The study, however, highlights how other factors fuel the process of not getting on and finding someone else. Among these factors, women have identified the fear and fact of violence. In the study by Bradshaw and Millar (1991), violence was a major or additional factor for one in five mothers splitting up from their partners. For many mothers, violence is not about one isolated incident, a momentary outburst that does not occur again. It is about a relationship in which a woman's sense of self and sense of survival is constantly under threat from the person who has assumed the place of lover and life-long companion in her life. As studies record, the majority of women escaping violent relationships have experienced the threat and use of violence against them for three years or more (Binny *et al.*, 1985; Pahl, 1985).

> He wanted something to eat. So I turned to go out of the bedroom and downstairs to the kitchen. He grabbed me at the top of the stairs yelling that I wasn't to walk away while he was talking to me. I tried to go downstairs. He pushed me. The stairs had two bends. I hit my head on the wall and rolled half-way down. Before I could stand up he kicked me. . . . Slowly I stood up and walked towards the bathroom. Then I felt him behind me. In panic I opened the front door and ran out of the house. . . . My nose was bleeding, my head was ringing and I was sure I wasn't able to hear properly, but above all was the pain in my chest. Every time I drew breath, I had a stabbing pain. . . . I leaned against the fence trying to make sense of what had just happened. Vowing not to go back into the house because he was going to be very angry. At least the kids had been asleep. The kids! I had forgotten the kids, I had to go back, there was no telling what he would do to them if I didn't. He had never hit them before but I lived in terror that he might one day. There was nowhere to go. My parents were long dead. There were no refuges I could go to and my neighbours didn't want to know. So fully aware that when I got back inside the house he was going to hit me again, I turned and walked back into the house.[5]

For many mothers the problems of finding accommodation is a

major deterrent to leaving a violent relationship (Pahl, 1985; Mama, 1989). For Black women, leaving a violent relationship can involve not only the risk of homelessness and a greater exposure to racism as women struggle to cope alone. It can also bring with it the threat of deportation because, in turning to the state for help, they can be forced to break the 'no recourse to public funds' clause in their immigration status (Mama, 1989; see Section 2.4).

Economic disadvantage marks out the pathways that women follow into lone motherhood. There is a clear class gradient in marriage breakdown. Divorce rates are higher among men in semi-skilled and unskilled occupations and, particularly, among unemployed men and younger men in these occupational groups. Divorce rates are significantly lower among men in social classes I and II, where age has little effect on the patterns of divorce. Among men in occupations which place them in social class I, one in every hundred can expect to divorce between the ages of 20 and 29. Among men in this age group in unskilled occupations, the divorce rate has been estimated to be 5.5 per 100, more than five times higher (Haskey, 1984).

Economic disadvantage is not only part of the cluster of factors that lead into lone motherhood; it is also a major consequence of lone motherhood. Most women find that their household income falls when their marriage ends (Chapter 4). For the majority, it is not earnings but social security benefits that provide them with the money they need to survive (Chapter 7).

> When I had to leave home with the children, it was as if I changed overnight from being a reasonably well off, secure middle class woman with a comfortable home and always enough money in my purse – to being sole financial support for three children without any means of providing that support. There we were out on our ear, no home, no money in the bank, instant total insecurity.[6]

> I'm much worse off (than when married). I'm in the same house. We are living on half the income. But I was very clear in my mind that the decision to separate was the decision to be much poorer.[7]

Material disadvantage also figures strongly in the lives of many single mothers. This is because single motherhood in Britain is linked to being young and working class. Most women under the age of 20 have their first baby outside marriage. The latest birth registration figures indicate that in this age group two in three women (66 per cent) having their first baby are unmarried. Among women in their early twenties, the proportion drops sharply to one in five (Office of Population Censuses and Surveys, 1991a). Vital registration provides only a partial picture of the class background of single mothers. For births outside marriage, the occupation of the baby's father is only recorded if he is present at the registration of the baby's birth (see Chapter 1). The data thus provide only an approximate guide to the class circumstances of single mothers. None the less, they suggest that women with partners in semi-skilled and unskilled manual occupations are more likely to have a baby outside marriage than women with partners in higher socioeconomic groups. Around 15 per cent of births registered by both parents in social classes I, II and IIINM are to parents who are not married. Such births make up over 25 per cent of births in social classes IIIM and IV, and 40 per cent of births in social class V (Office of Population Censuses and Surveys, 1991c).

Single women tend to face the same economic disadvantages as their partners. For many, it can be impossible to find and keep a job that provides enough to live on. Finding a home, too, can be a long, hard struggle (Simms and Smith, 1986; Clark, 1989). In her study of Black and White mothers, Ann Phoenix noted how poor job and housing prospects are part of the context in which women become pregnant when they are young and stay single after they become mothers (Phoenix, 1988; 1991).

> Oh yes, all the plans I'd had for myself went out the window. I was faced with a different sort of life to the one I'd thought about. I had to sit down and think about what I had to do, what I was going to come across. I knew that it wasn't going to be a bed of roses. I knew there would be hard times.

> I would have preferred not to, but now I don't mind. Maybe I could have gone out and found a career for myself, and maybe we could have got things a little more organised first. I'd like to have been a bit older but I don't think now it's going to make a lot of difference to my life. I will try not to make it.[8]

Having a baby outside marriage is strongly linked to being younger and poorer. However, not all single mothers are young and poor. The group also includes the increasing number of older women in more advantaged circumstances who are choosing to have children alone. While births outside marriage are more common among young women, the largest relative rise has occurred among women in the 25 to 34 age group. The number of births outside marriage among women in this group has trebled in the last decade (Jones, 1991). The category of single mothers also includes the small minority of women who have children within a lesbian relationship, adding to what has been described as a 'lesbian baby boom' in Britain and the United States (Levy, 1989; Walker, 1992).

> Megan was born in 1985, at home. Brenda did hold my hand during the delivery and for two and a half years she has been Megan's other mother. From the moment of her conception, I began coming out to Megan. She knows I am a lesbian in the same total, integrated way she knows I am her mother. Her discoveries will not be the sudden shock of a parent's revelation but the ongoing small bruises of a world which will not always accept me as Megan will.[9]

The increase in single motherhood and lone motherhood represent significant trends in family life in Britain. They are crosscut, however, by other experiences which are less often included in debates about 'the family'. One experience which runs through the family histories of many women is the process, and the aftermath, of immigrating to Britain.

2.4 Settling into Britain

Section 2.2 suggested that women's domestic lives in the late 1940s, 1950s and early 1960s were characterised by an orderly progression into early marriage and motherhood. What emerges from official statistics and survey data is the uniformity of women's lives during this period, both with respect to their relationships with men and the arrangements they made for the care of their children. However, personal stories point to a different reality. They highlight how, while many White women were building stable family units, many Black women were facing the enforced breakup of their families. In the two decades from

1945, thousands of women and men left their families to come to Britain at a time of acute labour shortage.

> We got a P & O liner from Bombay and I remember standing on the rail of the boat as it pulled away from India. That night my parents were crying and crying and India was getting smaller and smaller and smaller and all the lights were getting dimmer and dimmer, and I didn't really understand why they were crying. They were crying because they would never see her again. . . .
>
> When we docked at Tilbury we were taken to an immigrant hostel at the basement of a church near Selfridges. Men and women were separated and we slept in these iron cots. My dad walked all over London looking for somewhere to live but no one wanted coloureds or children. . . . The nearest (school) was St George's of Hanover Square, which was for all these posh kids from Mayfair. They were really racist to me. They used to pick on me all the time and I remember coming from a terrible day at school to sleep in these iron cots with people who were coughing and crying.[10]

The labour shortage was initially met by immigration from Eastern Europe and by continuing migration from Ireland. However, these sources quickly proved insufficient to meet the demand for labour. As a result, British employers sought to recruit newly arrived workers from the New Commonwealth. Through the 1950s, the pattern of immigration was closely tied to employment conditions in Britain, with the number of new workers rising and falling in line with job vacancies (Rose, 1969).

A few employers, including London Transport and the National Health Service, made arrangements with governments in the Caribbean for the direct recruitment of skilled workers and took initial responsibility for their accommodation. However, they were the exception: most of the new workers had to meet the costs of travelling to Britain and find their own accommodation when they arrived (Rose, 1969). Like those entering Britain through the direct recruitment schemes, the majority found their job opportunities were severely restricted. Black workers were 'replacement labour', filling the gaps at the bottom of the labour market and doing the jobs that White workers were becoming less inclined to do. Whatever their qualifications, Black workers found themselves disproportionately concentrated in low paid jobs in the unskilled and semi-skilled sectors of the job market and in the large industrial conurbations of Britain (Rose, 1969). It was a pattern that laid the basis for continuing occupational inequalities between Black and White workers in Britain. While the evidence points to some upward occupational mobility, ethnic minority employees are still clustered on the lower rungs of the job ladder (Brown, 1990). As the next chapter indicates, Black families, too, are still concentrated in the urban areas of Britain which have suffered most from unemployment and economic decline (Robinson, 1989).

> As a Black girl, I found myself in one of the lowest bands within Dick Sheppard Secondary School, London. Band five was where the majority of us were to be found. We were not expected to achieve any great heights academically. . . . Our parents worked for London Transport, the National Health Service, Fords, and British Rail; they worked as nurses, cooks, ticket collectors, guards and nursing auxiliaries doing shift hours. This meant that as girls we all had to take responsibilities for household chores: cooking, washing, looking after, and collecting younger sisters and brothers. Some of us had more responsibilities than others. Some of us had a bad time with our newly reunited families. Some girls had discovered they had families they did not know they had: older sisters, brothers, or stepfathers they hated. We talked and laughed, and cried together.[11]

Many African–Caribbean women came to Britain on their own, unaccompanied by parents, partners or children. They came as independent workers, looking for employment (Phizacklea, 1982). Among those travelling from the Indian subcontinent, the more usual pattern was for men to emigrate first, with partners and children hoping to join them later. For many Asian women, the timing of their arrival was influenced by the timing of the principal period of male emigration from India, Pakistan and Bangladesh, and by the increasingly restrictive regulations governing immigration control (Brah, 1992). Only among African–Asians, forced to leave Uganda under the Amin regime in the early 1970s, has there been a pattern of families migrating together (Diamond and Clarke, 1989). For other groups, the process of family unification has typically been a more protracted process. It is a process that is still continuing, particularly among Black families from Pakistan and Bangladesh. The relatively high ratio of men to women within these communities suggests that a substantial proportion of Bangladeshi and Pakistani families are still waiting to be reunited (Brah, 1992).

Legislation designed to limit Black immigration has made the process of reunification progressively more difficult. Through the 1960s and 1970s, legislation had a particular effect on Black women seeking to build families in Britain. Laws and rules governing immigration were framed around the assumption that women were the dependents of men, with the result that women had fewer rights than men to be joined by spouses and children (Bhabha *et al.*, 1985). Specific regulations, too, worked against women wanting to be joined by relatives. For example, regulations passed in the 1960s governing the admission of children into Britain stipulated that they could only join a lone parent if the parent had 'sole responsibility' for the child's upbringing. It was a rule that has particularly affected single women from the Caribbean. Many had left their children with kin, making it very difficult to prove that they had sole responsibility for their upbringing (Bhabha *et al.*, 1985).

The last major piece of legislation, the 1988 Immigration Act, placed further barriers in the way of Black women wanting to join, and be joined by, their families. The Act withdrew the automatic right of Commonwealth citizens to be joined by their spouse and children. The right is now a conditional one and depends on their ability to accommodate and to maintain themselves and their dependents with 'no recourse to public funds' (Gordon, 1991). The term 'public funds' covers income support, housing benefit, family credit and housing under Part III of the 1985 Housing Act, which relates to housing for homeless people (Child Poverty Action Group, 1992).

The 'no recourse to public funds' condition has a long history in Britain immigration policy. It was, for example, incorporated into legislation designed to control Jewish immigration at the turn of the century and has been a central plank of policies relating to the settlement of Black families in Britain (Cohen, 1985). What the 1988 Act has done, however, is to stipulate that 'people who have lived here for years, and who have worked and paid taxes, are now allowed to be joined by their families from abroad only on condition that they do not claim benefits for them and can provide them with accommodation' (Gordon, 1991, pp.80–1). Underlining the racism of the Act, these conditions do not apply to other people lawfully settled in Britain, including European Community (EC) citizens (Gordon, 1991; Child Poverty Action Group, 1992). Combined with earlier restrictions, their effect has been to move reunification beyond the reach of a significant minority of Black families in Britain.

> (Some of) my children were not allowed to stay here. These children were born here and the Home Office sent them back to Pakistan last year.

> It took me six years to bring my wife. I would like to bring my mother for a permanent stay but can't due to immigration rules. She can only come as a visitor. My application for British nationality has been refused.

> I miss my wife and children who cannot be with me. . . . We worry about attacks on our women and children. . . . I had this sort of interview before in London when I asked for help to bring in my family, but nobody did anything.[12]

2.5 Family patterns among Black and White women

Personal stories record how difficult it has been for many Black families to settle in Britain. Official statistics paint a more clinical picture of the impact of labour migration on family life. Because it was predominantly young adults who made the long journey to Britain during the 1950s, 1960s and early 1970s, Britain's Black minority groups have a youthful age structure that stands in marked contrast to the ageing population profile found among the majority White populations. This demographic profile is reflected, in turn, in the patterns of household composition, with a larger proportion of households containing dependent children among Black minority ethnic groups. Data from the General Household Survey, summarised in Figure 2.3, suggest that 29 per cent of households with a White head of household contain children under 16. In households with an African–Caribbean head, the proportion is 46 per cent; in Indian-headed households, it is nearly 60 per cent. Among Pakistani and Bangladeshi households, the proportion rises to 78 per cent (Office of Population Censuses and Surveys, 1991a).

While most White women have children in the country in

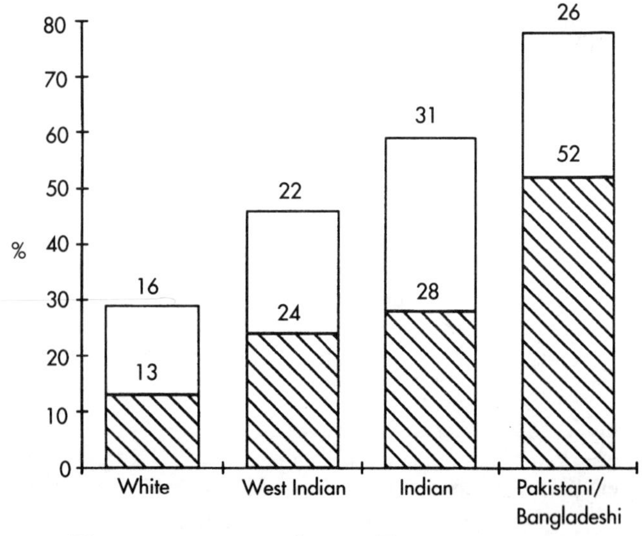

Figure 2.3 Proportion of households with children under 16, by ethnic group of head of household, Britain, 1987–9 combined.

Source: Office of Population Censuses and Surveys (1991a), derived from Table 2.54.

which they were born, African–Caribbean and Asian mothers are much more likely to have a birthplace outside the United Kingdom. Table 2.1 describes the birthplace of people in Britain aged both under 25 and 25 and over. It suggests that all but a small minority of the adult White population in both these age groups were born in the United Kingdom. Among African–Caribbean people over the age of 25, 80 per cent are non-UK born; among Asian people, the proportion rises to almost 100 per cent. In contrast, children born to African–Caribbean and Asian parents, like children born to White parents, are typically born in the United Kingdom.

In trying to build a family life in Britain, women and their partners have worked to express their different cultural and religious traditions. In many Asian communities, marriage is the lynchpin of the kinship system and the setting in which children are expected to be born. Births outside marriage go against these values and the proportion of births to unmarried Asian women is,

Table 2.1 Place of birth and ethnic identity, Britain, 1987–9 combined.

	% born in the UK	
	under 25	25 and over
White	98	96
West Indian/Guyanese	96	20
Indian	76	2
Pakistani/Bangladeshi	70	1

Source: Office of Population Censuses and Surveys (1991a), Table 2.51. (Reproduced by permission of G.H.S. Unit, Social Survey Division, OPCS)

in consequence, very low. Among Indian-born women, 2 per cent of births in 1990 were to single women. Among Pakistani and Bangladeshi women, it was 1 per cent. In contrast, the proportion among UK-born women was 30 per cent (Jones, 1991).

Family units in Asian communities have tended to encompass a wider range of relatives than White families. More mothers care for their children in households in which three rather than two generations live together. Data from the Labour Force Survey suggest that family units containing parents, children and other household members are more common among Indian, Pakistani and Bangladeshi households. These family units make up approximately one in ten Asian households; among White, African–Caribbean, African and Chinese-headed households, the proportion is less than one in forty (Haskey, 1989a).

For African–Caribbean women, too, cultural traditions are expressed in family structures. Marriage is not the gateway to adulthood and the guardian of family honour that it is in many Asian households. Marriage is more likely to be postponed until a man can provide some financial security, with children often born within non-cohabiting relationships (Phizacklea, 1982). As noted earlier, it is a pattern found among White women, too. When their partners are unlikely to find a job that pays enough to support a family, young African–Caribbean and White women may choose to stay single and not to cohabit (Phoenix, 1991). Compared to Asian women, a relatively high proportion of children born to African–Caribbean and White women are born outside marriage (Jones, 1991).

> In the West Indies, where I come from, people don't get married just because a woman's pregnant. In many cases, a man and woman will get married after they've had children. In my situation, the appropriate time for us to have got married would have been after he qualified. Similarly, in the West Indies it is things other than children that determine when the right time is to get married. For most of the West Indian people that I know, marriage isn't a big thing in the way it is for some White people. My mother says it's better to live together and be happy, than to be married and unhappy.[13]

Cultural expectations about how women should lead their lives are reflected in the pathways that Black and White women take through adult life. Women in Asian-headed households are very unlikely to be bringing up their children as lone mothers. The patterns uncovered in the Labour Force Survey are summarised in Table 2.2. They suggest that well over 90 per cent of mothers in these households are married. Among women in Chinese-headed households, the proportion is higher still. Lone motherhood is more common among White, African and African–Caribbean women. One in eight (13 per cent) of White households with dependent children are female-headed; among African households, one in four (27 per cent) are headed by a

Table 2.2 Family types by ethnic group.

Ethnic group of head of family	Lone mother (%)	Lone father (%)	Married couples (%)
Chinese	(1)	(0)	98
Arab	(4)	(1)	95
Indian	6	(1)	94
Pakistani	6	(2)	92
Bangladeshi	(5)	(3)	92
White	13	2	85
African	27	(2)	70
West Indian	44	5	51
All	13	2	85

Notes:
1. Dependent children are persons under 16 or 16 to 18 and in full-time education.
2. Bracketed estimates are based on sample sizes of 30 or less.

Source: Haskey (1991), Table 4. (Reproduced by permission of the Information Division, OPCS)

woman. In African–Caribbean households with children, the data suggest that 44 per cent are headed by women (Haskey, 1991a).

The patterns summarised in Table 2.2 reflect cultural diversity among mothers. But they also reflect cultural change. Black women, like White women, are not the passive carriers of culture, constructing domestic lives in ways prescribed by tradition. Instead, Black and White women describe how they negotiate the values that shape their identities (Phoenix, 1988; Bhachu, 1991; Drury, 1991). A study of Sikh women recorded how women are challenging the sexual division of labour in their families, moving away from a three-generational household structure towards nuclear family units with more egalitarian relationships between men and women (Bhachu, 1991). Other studies have noted, too, how women are changing cultures as they live them. For example, in Brah's study of Asian and White adolescent boys and girls and their parents, the dominant ideology was one in which women took responsibility for the housework and childcare. The strongest opposition to this sexual division of labour came from Asian girls, with half of her sample insisting that housework should be shared on an equal basis (Brah, 1992).

> It's going to be different. For a start, we will have a social life, we'll go to parties and discos. My Dad goes to the pub but he never takes Mum. I'm not having that. He's not going to go out and leave me at home. . . . I'll treat my sons and daughters the same. My son will have to do the housework and my daughter will be allowed more freedom than me. The sons will have to come home in the evenings at the same time as the girls. More equality, that's it.[14]

For Black women, as for White women, achieving more equality in their relationships with their children assumes that they are able to find a place for them to live together with them. Implicit in the notion of a household is the existence of a home. It is to the question of housing that the next chapter turns.

Notes

1. Walker (1992), pp.215–16.
2. Taking Liberties Collective (1989), p.32.

3. Two stepmothers quoted in Hughes (1991), pp.67 and 52.
4. Walker, (1992), pp.211–12.
5. Taking Liberties Collective (1989), p.23.
6. Taking Liberties Collective (1989), p.4.
7. Lone mother quoted in Graham, (1985), p.121.
8. Two expectant mothers, aged 18 and 19, quoted in Phoenix (1991), p.96.
9. Cathy in MacPike (1989), p.5.
10. Salvat (1989), pp.93–4.
11. Williams (1988), p.153.
12. Asian middle-aged and older people quoted in Fenton (1985), pp.12–13.
13. Jules (1992), p.76.
14. Young Sikh woman quoted in Drury (1991), p.397.

CHAPTER 3

FINDING A HOME

3.1 Introduction

The last chapter explored some of the different kinds of family lives that women build for themselves and their children. However, home lives turn not only on domestic relationships: they have a material dimension too. Making a home means having a safe and secure place in which to bring up children.

This chapter begins by reviewing the recent changes in housing policy, as a backcloth against which to set women's experiences of trying to find decent accommodation for themselves and their children. The central sections of the chapter examine different dimensions of housing inequality among women with children. The sections look in turn at women's access to housing, the increase in homelessness among families with children and the role of council housing in accommodating mothers who cannot buy themselves out of this residual housing sector. The chapter concludes by considering some of the evidence which links poor health among mothers and their children to the poor housing in which they live.

3.2 Housing policy

From 1945 to the early 1970s, Britain followed a 'twin-track' housing policy. It was a policy in which both owner-occupied (private) and council-rented (public) housing was encouraged. While the public sector was designed to accommodate a broad cross-section of the population, it was recognised that it had a particular role to play in the provision of social housing, housing for people who were disadvantaged in the commercial market. New houses were built by local authorities and new town corporations, while owner-occupation increased through a combination of rising real incomes, tax relief on mortgage interest and the expansion of credit facilities. The result was a significant growth in both council-rented housing and owner-occupation and a decline in privately rented accommodation through the 1950s, 1960s and 1970s (Hills and Mullings, 1990). By the late 1970s, over half (55 per cent) of Britain's homes were owner-occupied, with nearly a third (32 per cent) rented from local authorities and new towns.

The twin-track framework, however, was giving way. Through the late 1970s and 1980s, housing policy was shunted onto a single track through the stimulation of home ownership and the withdrawal of support for council housing (Ginsberg, 1992). Owner-occupation was encouraged by maintaining tax relief on mortgage interest which, by the end of the 1980s, represented three-quarters of total public expenditure on housing, including housing benefit (Hills and Mullings, 1990). Owner-occupation was also supported through increasing the opportunities for council house tenants to buy their homes at discounted prices, enshrined in the Right to Buy measures of the 1980 Housing Act. The homes lost to the council sector have been predominantly houses with gardens on suburban estates. Because most of the tenants on these estates are White, the effect of Right to Buy measures has been to widen racial inequalities in housing (Ginsberg, 1992).

Under the single-track policy of the 1980s and 1990s, the social housing function of local authorities has been shed. Over the last decade, housing associations have been encouraged to take on this role, but in the context of declining capital investment in housing (Hills and Mullings, 1990). The number of new housing association homes completed each year has fallen across the last decade, at a time when fewer new council homes have been built. The number of new homes built by local authorities and new towns fell from 146,000 a year in the mid-1970s, to less than 19,000 by the end of the 1980s, a fall of nearly 90 per cent (Hills and Mullings, 1990). At the same time, local authority rents rose substantially in real terms and, as a result, tenants found themselves spending a larger proportion of their income on their rent.

The changes in housing policy and provision have occurred against a backdrop of wider social and economic change. Patterns of family life in Britain are diversifying (see Chapter 2). Recent decades have also witnessed a large-scale restructuring of employment in Britain, with declining job opportunities in the old industrial areas and conurbations (see Chapter 6). These factors have combined to widen inequalities in women's access to decent housing for themselves and their children. Specifically, they are affecting women's access to tenured housing and are increasing the number of mothers caring for children in temporary accommodation. Council housing is increasingly becoming a residual sector for those who do not have the money to buy into owner-occupation.

These interlocking aspects of housing inequality are explored in turn in the sections below.

3.3 Access to housing

Today two-thirds (66 per cent) of homes in Britain are owner-occupied (Office of Population Censuses and Surveys, 1991a). The growth in owner-occupation reflects the long-term trend away from the private-rented sector. It also reflects the transfer of dwellings out of the council sector since 1980.

Access to the owner-occupied sector depends on income. It is those on higher incomes who take out mortgages and exercise the Right to Buy their council homes (Hills and Mullings, 1990). Through the 1980s and 1990s, an increasing number of homebuyers have faced problems meeting the costs of their mortgage repayments. In 1979, around 8000 homeowners were more than six months in arrears on their repayments. By the middle of 1991, the figure was over 150,000, nearly 20 times higher. By mid-1992, 300,000 households were at least six months in arrears. The increase in arrears has gone hand in hand with a sharp rise in the number of repossessions. In 1979, 2500 properties were taken into possession, by 1991, the figure was over 75,000 (Coles, 1990; Skellington, 1993).

While an increasing number of households are being forced out of owner-occupation, there has been a sharp reduction in the supply of rented accommodation. Through the 1980s, the number of homes for rent fell by over a million (Raynsford, 1989). London has been particularly hard hit by the increasing shortage of rented accommodation (Greve, 1991). As the supply of homes for renting has fallen, so council-house waiting lists have lengthened and the number of households accepted as homeless by local authorities has increased. Between 1978 and 1990, the number of officially recognised homeless households in England trebled to 150,000 (Hills and Mullings, 1990; Central Statistical Office, 1992).

Officially homeless households are those defined as homeless according to the 1977 Housing (Homeless Persons) Act (now Part III of the 1985 Housing Act). Local authorities are obliged to rehouse people who are, or are likely to be, without accommodation and who have a 'priority need'. People in priority need include pregnant women, households with children and those who are vulnerable because of old age, mental illness or physical disability. Women escaping domestic violence do not have a statutory right to accommodation, and women without children who leave home because of domestic violence are not normally accepted as a priority group within the terms of Part III of the 1985 Housing Act (Sexty, 1990).

Because most single and childless people are excluded from the rehousing provisions of the 1985 Housing Act, official statistics significantly underestimate the scale of homelessness in Britain. It is, as Nick Raynsford (1989) observes, a chilling reminder of the inadequacy of housing statistics that most of those sleeping rough do not feature in the official homelessness figures.

The growth in official and unofficial homelessness has been identified as part of a wider 'access crisis', in which increasing numbers of people are finding it impossible to gain access to the formal housing market (Kleinman and Whitehead, 1988). Significant among those affected by this access crisis are mothers searching for decent housing in which to build a home for their children. Housing problems are often particularly acute for disabled women, who rely heavily on the public sector for housing that supports independent living (see Section 3.5) (J. Morris,

1990). Young mothers, disabled and non-disabled, are also facing increasing problems in finding a place to live. In one study of mothers aged under 20, nearly half were living with parents or relatives after the birth of their babies and not in independent households of their own. Four in ten were living in overcrowded conditions (a density of one or more persons per room), a proportion four times higher than the national average (Simms and Smith, 1986). Not surprisingly, housing was identified by the mothers as a significant cause of the depression and anxiety that many experienced (Simms and Smith).

> . . . I hate living in this flat. I can't stand it, but I can't get a council flat . . . So at the moment we're waiting because the council might be compulsorily purchasing the building, so, crossed fingers, we might actually end up being council tenants. . . . Well, it's the room really, 'cos Benjamin shares the bedroom with us. Also, as you can see, there's not a bit of privacy, you know, you can't switch off from Benjamin at all, you know. He can't be in a separate part, he's there all the time. You can't turn the telly on too loud because it might wake him up or whatever. But, I mean we manage reasonably well, y'know. I only lose me cool every now and then (laughs) apart from that we sort of work it out okay.[1]

Like young mothers trying to set up homes, Black and White women trying to leave relationships face particular housing problems. Relationship breakdown often involves a change in housing circumstances for one or both partners, and is a significant cause of rent and mortgage arrears and homelessness (Kemp, 1989). Women's homelessness is linked, particularly, to the experience of violence in domestic relationships (see Chapter 2).

> I left my husband. I had a flat in Putney. I left him because he started to become violent. . . . I'd been with him about ten years, married for about four. Finally, I couldn't stand any more so I left him. . . . not only am I pregnant now, but I haven't got a job. So I moved in with my sister. And my sister couldn't put up with me; she only has a two-bedroom flat. She's got two children of her own. There was her and her boyfriend, she was pregnant again, and she had my mum living with her. So it was a great strain to

> live with my sister. Well, in the end I went along to Lewisham Council. Lewisham said they weren't taking any responsibility, that I should be under Wandsworth. So I've been in bed and breakfast now a year . . .[2]

As the account above suggests, the accommodation changes that follow separation and divorce typically involve moving down-market, into poorer housing (Bradshaw and Millar, 1991). Living with relatives and living in crisis accommodation are woven into the housing experiences of many lone mothers.

> Friends who have known me for a long time say that I started at the top and have worked my way down! I didn't want to be dependent on him (ex-husband) and it was agreed that the house would be sold. I got half the sum and an extra sum which paid for most of this house. I have moved from one of the 'better' neighbourhoods of Birmingham to one of the poorer areas. I see it as the price I pay for independence.[3]

Restricted access to the housing market is linked to restricted access to good quality housing in materially advantaged neighbourhoods. The patterns found among lone mothers and Black mothers (groups which are not, of course, mutually exclusive) illustrate how social divisions are meshed into the housing circumstances of Britain's families. Census data suggest that one-parent families are over-represented in the metropolitan authorities: in Greater London, Greater Manchester and Merseyside, and under-represented in the suburban and rural areas of Britain (Haskey, 1991b). Within the metropolitan areas, one-parent families are concentrated in the inner city cores, areas that have been hardest hit by the movement of jobs and people out of Britain's major conurbations. The highest concentrations of one-parent families are found in the London boroughs, including Lambeth, Hackney and Hammersmith (Haskey, 1991b).

A similar spatial patterning is evident among Black families. The conurbations, and Greater London in particular, have provided the major areas of residence for Britain's Black minority populations. While 9 per cent of the White population live in Greater London, the General Household Survey suggests that 44 per cent of the Indian population of Britain do so. Three in five (60 per cent) African–Caribbean people live in Greater London. Of the other conurbations, the West Midlands and West Yorkshire are also significant areas of Black settlement, particularly for people from Pakistan and Bangladesh (Office of Population Censuses and Surveys, 1991a). Within these conurbations, analyses of the census data suggest that Black families are under-represented in neighbourhoods which are materially advantaged: in suburban and rural neighbourhoods with high levels of employment, owner-occupation and car-ownership. They are over-represented in poorer urban areas, with high rates of unemployment and low car-ownership (Robinson, 1989).

> We live in this dump because I couldn't find nothing else. It's very difficult to find places to rent with children. Most landlords just don't want to know and those that do charge more for places they couldn't let to other people. They take advantage because they know that you couldn't find another place. So I'm in no position to stick up for myself and complain about the damp and the smell from the drain.[4]

The disadvantages that Black families, and Black and White mothers caring for children alone, face in the housing market are reflected in the patterns of homelessness in Britain. These patterns are the focus of the next section.

3.4 Homeless families

Reflecting the priority categories laid down in the 1977 Housing Act, the vast majority of those accepted by local authorities as homeless and found accommodation are pregnant women and families with children (Central Statistical Office, 1992). Figure 3.1 indicates that, in 1990, 78 per cent of the homeless households who were found accommodation by local authorities fell into one of these two categories.

An increasing proportion of expectant mothers and parents with children who are recognised as officially homeless are being placed in temporary accommodation. Temporary accommodation includes bed and breakfast hotels, short-life tenancies, women's refuges and hostels.

> I was here (in the hotel) before the baby was born, two weeks before. I was so frightened, so alone. I had no transport, nothing. I sat here and cried my eyes out the whole night, I felt so alone. Then, later when I went into labour, I didn't even know I was in labour, I just waited and then went to the hospital and said I was

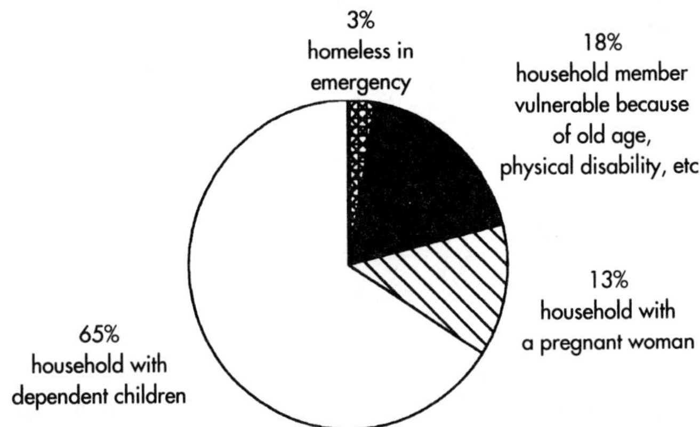

Figure 3.1 Homeless households found accommodation by local authorities by priority need category, Britain, 1990.

Note: Households for whom local authorities accepted responsibility to secure accommodation under the Housing Act 1985 which defines 'priority need'. Data for Wales include some households given advice and assistance only.
Source: Central Statistical Office (1992), derived from Table 8.12.

> terrified. I came back five days after the birth, and the first few days were terrible, you want to show off, you know, but you haven't got the space, the organisation, you're just ashamed of where you are and that you haven't got a home for your child.[5]

The evidence suggests that the majority of households in temporary accommodation are households with children, and a large proportion are headed by lone mothers. In a recent Department of Environment study of 1000 households in temporary accommodation, 40 per cent were single-parent households (Thomas and Niner, 1989). Mothers can expect to spend 33 weeks in temporary accommodation before being rehoused.

> When I first went into bed and breakfast, they stuck me up 72 stairs with a baby and a buggy and shopping. I was in a tiny little room which wasn't even six foot by eight foot. After many months of complaining . . . they moved me right downstairs into the basement. It wasn't too bad, apart from people chucking dirty, soiled nappies into the basement. Every morning when I opened my window, I've got a dirty nappy looking at me. The kitchens are

> atrocious, absolutely filthy downstairs, so that I can't cook in that sort of condition. I used to buy food from takeaways and things like that, but my son got ill. He went into bed and breakfast when he was about four months old; he's now about fourteen months old. I've got so many problems with him. Because he's not on a proper diet, he still wakes up of a night time, he very rarely sleeps. Now he's walking but he's still very, very small for his age.[6]

'Race' is also deeply structured into the patterns of official and unofficial homelessness in Britain. A survey in Brent found that the number of African–Caribbean people who were officially accepted as homeless was three times that of White people (Bonnerjea and Lawton, 1987). There is also evidence that Black families are offered temporary accommodation inferior to that offered to White families and spend longer in it (Ginsberg, 1992). As the latest group of newcomers to Britain, Bangladeshi families have suffered disproportionately from the squeeze on public sector housing and the restrictions on recourse to public funds imposed by immigration legislation (Miller, 1990). Evidence presented to the House of Commons Home Affairs Committee (1986) on Bangladeshi families suggested that 90 per cent of those classified as homeless in Tower Hamlets in the mid-1980s were Bangladeshi and they made up over 80 per cent of the homeless families placed in bed and breakfast accommodation.

Temporary accommodation often means substandard accommodation. A government survey reported that about half of the properties housing homeless people were below an acceptable standard (Thomas and Niner, 1989). The report also found that over three-quarters (76 per cent) of local authority hostels and over 90 per cent of hotels were substandard or poor based on such measures as overcrowding, amenities and means of escape in case of fire.

> My family came to England in 1975 or '76. My dad was here, we came to join him (from Bangladesh). . . . I was living with my mother, and I got pregnant with my first child. It's a very small flat, near Victoria. When she was born, I had to go to the Homeless because there was no room for me. When I first went there, I went straight from the hospital. They put me in the first hotel and it was terrible; really like an attic; the window was broken. . . . There were plenty of cockroaches. I was terrified of them. I used to be out most of the day, I used to come home just to sleep. When I used to go into the room I used to think, this is a

prison. I used to cry to myself. I think people living in a hotel long-term probably go mental. I find it myself, and I'm a very capable woman.[7]

3.5 Living in council housing

Public sector housing is increasingly becoming a residual housing sector, occupied by households without the income to buy a home of their own. Rather than accommodating a broad social mix, as intended in the twin-track policies of the post-war decades, council accommodation houses those who are struggling against disadvantage. Council tenants live on the margins of the labour market. Over 60 per cent of the heads of council households are economically inactive and, among those in paid work, incomes are less than 60 per cent of the average for all economically active heads of households (Office of Population Censuses and Surveys, 1991a). Council homes are increasingly female-headed homes. While one quarter (25 per cent) of all households in Britain are female-headed, over 40 per cent of council-rented households have a female head.

It is older women living alone and lone mothers who predominate among these female-headed households. As Figure 3.2 indicates, lone-parent households are concentrated in the rented sector while two-parent households are concentrated in the owner-occupied sector. Within the rented sector, it is council accommodation that provides homes for the majority (54 per cent) of Britain's one-parent families. The role of public housing was underlined in the Bradshaw and Millar study of 1400 lone parents. Reflecting the class differences in marriage breakdown and single motherhood, more lone parents came from local authority housing. Becoming a lone parent was associated with a change of address for the majority (58 per cent) of their respondents and most of those who moved house, passed through or were eventually housed by local authorities (Bradshaw and Millar, 1991).

The patterns mapped out in Figure 3.2 match those found among parents caring for non-disabled children. Families with a disabled child, however, are less likely to be owner–occupiers than other families with children. In the late 1980s, 76 per cent of two-parent families were owner–occupiers: the evidence from the OPCS surveys of disability suggest that the proportion of

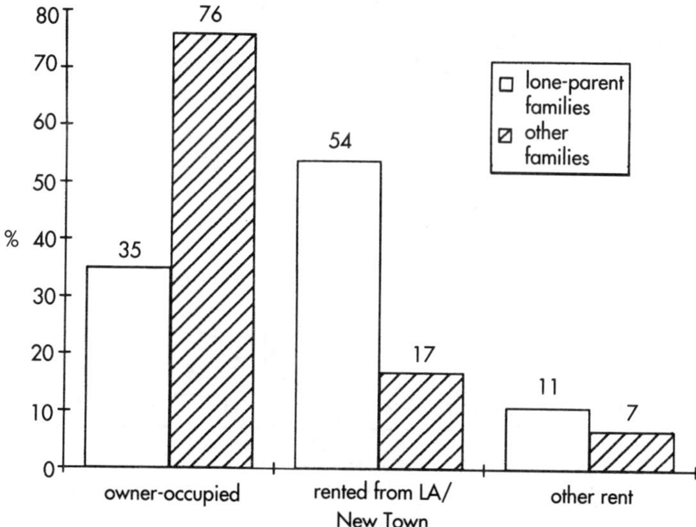

Figure 3.2 Housing tenure of lone-parent families and other families with dependent children, Britain, 1988–9.

Note: Dependent children are persons under 16 or aged 16 to 18 and in full-time education, in the family unit and living in the household. *Source:* Office of Population Censuses and Surveys (1991a), derived from Table 2.41.

homeowners among two-parent families with a disabled child was under 60 per cent. Similarly, the national evidence on lone mothers suggests that 54 per cent rent from the local authority: among lone parents caring for disabled children, the proportion is 77 per cent (Smyth and Robus, 1989). These patterns of housing tenure are summarised in Figure 3.3.

Council housing is the sector in which most disabled adults live (J. Morris, 1990). As Morris notes, this is partly because of their generally lower incomes. It is also because most housing which is purpose-built or adapted for disabled people is owned by local authorities. Among disabled parents, too, the evidence suggests that the public sector is a much more important source of housing than it is among non-disabled parents. Data from the OPCS surveys of disability, reproduced in Figure 3.4, relate to the housing tenure of disabled parents who are householders. It is

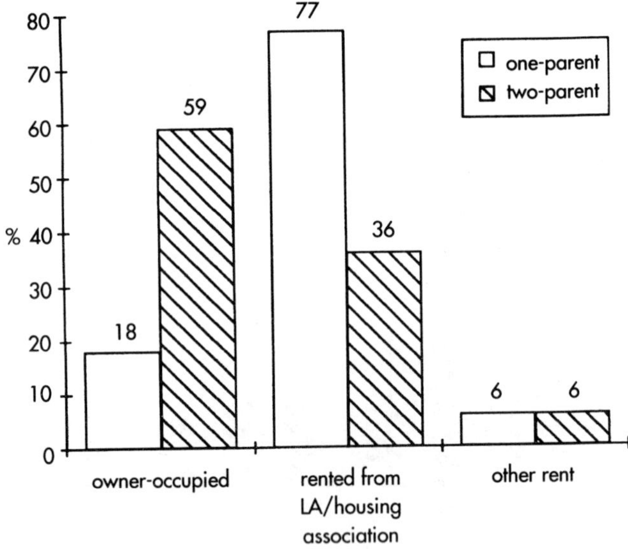

Figure 3.3 Housing tenure of households with a disabled child, Britain, 1985.

Source: Smyth and Robus (1989), derived from Table 2.5.

likely, therefore, to reflect the tenure patterns among fathers rather than mothers in two-parent households and mothers rather than fathers in one-parent households. It indicates that, compared to the general population of married and cohabiting parents, disabled parents who head a two-parent household are much more likely to be council tenants (42 per cent compared with 17 per cent among two-parent families as a whole). Among disabled lone parents, over seven in ten (73 per cent) are council tenants compared with five in ten (54 per cent) of lone parents in general (see Figures 3.2 and 3.4).

Public sector housing reflects the divisions of 'race' as well as those of class, gender and disability. Local authorities provide homes for a large proportion of African–Caribbean families. Data from the General Household Survey suggest that African–Caribbean households are significantly more likely to rent their accommodation from local authorities (42 per cent) than White households (25 per cent), Pakistani and Bangladeshi households (17 per cent) or Indian households (8 per cent) (Office of Population Censuses and Surveys, 1991a). A complex of factors

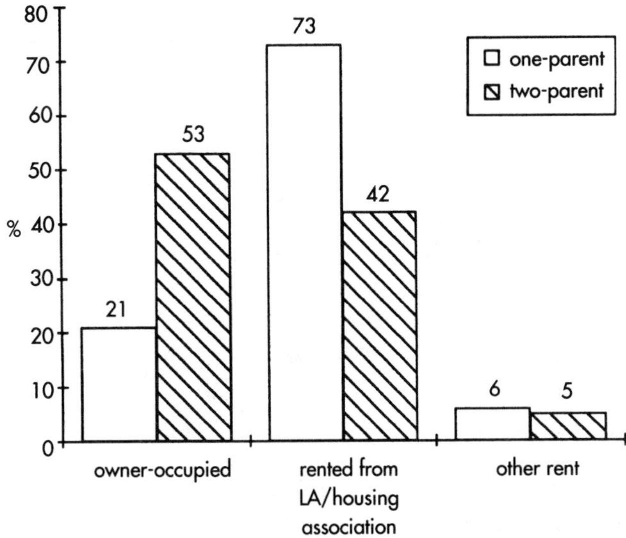

Figure 3.4 Housing tenure of disabled adults who are householders in households with children, Britain, 1985.

Source: Martin and White (1988), derived from Table 2.14.

are woven into these different patterns, including the preference of many Asian families to own the homes they live in. However, housing preferences are not the only influences at work. Studies have recorded how the allocation procedures governing access to public sector housing have discriminated, directly and indirectly, against African–Caribbean and Asian households.

One major study highlighted the formal procedures which restrict the access of Black applicants seeking council housing. The criteria relating to length of residence, the disqualification of owner-occupiers and the rejection of applications from joint families worked against Asian applicants particularly, while the less favourable treatment of unmarried cohabiting couples was a major obstacle for African–Caribbean applicants. The study also highlighted the informal working practices which meant that applicants were 'matched' to properties and areas on the basis of their 'race', gender and class characteristics (Henderson and Karn, 1987).

While Henderson and Karn's research was conducted in the 1970s, their conclusions have been confirmed by more recent studies. A study of council housing in the London boroughs of Wandsworth and Southwark pointed to longer waiting periods among Black women than among White women. The study also found that White women were more likely to live in semi-detached and terraced housing, while Black women were more likely to live in flats, and on the upper floors of high-rise blocks (Rao, 1990). These differences were reflected in the patterns of council housing among women with children. For example, among the White women with three or more children in the study, 65 per cent were living in one-bedroomed flats or maisonettes; the proportion among Black and minority ethnic women was 90 per cent.

> I don't think it's just chance that there are so many Black families in this block, the council puts us here. Lots of them are lone parents too. I don't think it's good to put us all together like this because the block gets a bad reputation and just because we are alone with our kids doesn't mean we all get on. But I do have some good mates round here.[8]

3.6 Poor housing and poor health

A house provides the physical context in which domestic relationships are built and lived out. It is the place in which women experience what it is to be a mother and have responsibilities for the health of children. As the accounts included in this chapter illustrate, women recognise that the physical environment of the home affects how they feel about themselves and their lives. They recognise, too, that poor and poorly designed housing spells danger for their children (Mayall, 1986). It brings with it hazards which mean that children must be constantly restrained and mothers must be constantly vigilant.

> The flat's too restricted – he's no room to play and he loves climbing. And if there was a fire, how would we get out? It worries me terribly. My Nan was in a fire, she was very badly burned. I try to keep him out of the kitchen while I'm cooking, because he can reach up to things. But if I shut him out, I can't see what he's up to.

> He's too confined. He's not getting enough exercise. It'll be worse when he's older. I won't be able to let him run around outside because it's a rough area, and the people – it's like any council estate. The windows are very bad. They're low down and they've got loose handles – he'll soon be able to open them. He can reach up to them now. I have to keep the windows shut – it's a problem in these small rooms. It gets very hot. I have to watch him, all the time. Keep telling him – it's wrong, mustn't do that.[9]

The relationship between poor housing and poor health was underlined in a recent study of households with children in Glasgow, Edinburgh and London (Hunt *et al.*, 1988). Reflecting the design of the study, a large proportion of the parents and children lived in low-income households where there was no-one in employment. It was typically the mother rather than the father who was interviewed about their health and the health of children in the household, while the presence and severity of dampness and mould was assessed by surveyors. The survey pointed to a gradient of physical ill-health with the proportion of adults reporting a range of symptoms, including nausea, coughs, blocked nose and high blood pressure, increasing in line with the levels of damp and mould in the home (Hunt *et al.*, 1988).

A similar gradient in children's health also emerged. Children in homes with high damp and mould scores were reported to have higher rates of respiratory and gastrointestinal symptoms, aches and pains, and fever than children in dry and mould-free homes (Platt *et al.*, 1989). For example, the proportion of children with headaches rose from 12 per cent of those in damp-free homes to 30 per cent of those in homes judged to be very damp (Hunt *et al.*, 1988). The association between damp and mouldy housing and a child's poor health status has been confirmed in other studies (Strachan, 1988).

Poor housing conditions were not only associated with symptoms of physical ill-health. The survey found a similarly strong association with mothers' and children's emotional well-being. Mothers living in households assessed to be damp and mouldy were more likely to report such symptoms as tiredness, 'bad nerves', headaches and feeling low. Mothers living in homes that they assessed to be cold, noisy and in poor repair also reported more emotional distress than those living without these problems (Hunt, 1990). Children growing up in homes which were damp were more likely to be described by their mothers as irritable, tired and with a poor appetite. They were also more likely to be described as unhappy.

Other studies have confirmed the links between poor housing and emotional distress among women. For example, a study of 800 families in Waltham Forest found that mothers with preschool children living in council-rented accommodation were more likely to be depressed than mothers in owner-occupied accommodation (Richman *et al.*, 1982). This study, like others, pointed to higher rates of depression among mothers living in flats above ground level and in tower blocks (Littlewood and Tinker, 1981).

> It's the house. It just gets on my nerves. We can't get another one until they pull it down. It's damp, we've no hot water, no bath and the toilet's outside. It's just this place.

> It's too cramped. There's five of us in one bedroom at the moment. He has to sleep in his carry cot as I don't have enough room to put his proper cot up.[10]

The links between housing difficulties and emotional distress figured strongly in Brown and Harris' research into the social origins of depression among White women. On the basis of information collected from over 700 women, they identified a set of difficulties and experiences which provoked depression. Difficulties were only included if they were markedly unpleasant, were long term (of at least two years' duration) and involved problems other than health. Housing was the major long term difficulty faced by women. For half the women with difficulties, their problems were related to their housing: severe overcrowding, lack of amenities, noise and insecurity of tenure. The researchers concluded that major housing problems 'are highly associated with chronic psychiatric conditions' and that such difficulties 'play a definite aetiological role in depression' (Brown and Harris, 1978, pp.199 and 276).

> . . . there's no door to the bedroom, there's no privacy whatsoever and consequently 'cos there's no door there you can't put him down like most people do at 9 o'clock in his own little room. You try putting him down and he just screams his head off. Midnight it was last night and it has been for about the last week. . . . also,

> when I'm on nights most of the week I know I have to get up for him in the morning, but on Fridays his dad gets up and gets him breakfast and I should by rights be able to sleep through but it's impossible.[11]

Poor housing in materially deprived neighbourhoods provides the setting in which an increasing number of women are working to bring up their children. Their experiences of caring at home and for their families are the focus of the next two chapters.

Notes

1. Mother quoted in Fulop (1992), p.188.
2. Lone mother quoted in Miller (1990), p.38.
3. Divorced mother quoted in Crow and Hardey (1991), p.55.
4. Lone mother quoted in Crow and Hardey (1991), pp.59–60.
5. Mother quoted in Bonnerjea and Lawton (1987), p.38–9.
6. Lone mother quoted in Miller (1990), p.39.
7. Married mother quoted in Miller (1990), pp.79–80; 81.
8. Lone mother quoted in Crow and Hardey (1991), p.62.
9. Two mothers interviewed in Mayall (1986), pp.60–1.
10. Mothers under 20 quoted in Simms and Smith (1986), pp.70 and 62.
11. Mother quoted in Fulop (1992), p.187.

CHAPTER 4

BEING A MOTHER

4.1 Introduction

The previous two chapters have explored the domestic settings in which women become mothers. They have highlighted the increasing diversity in patterns of childbearing and childrearing, a diversity structured by inequalities in women's access to housing for themselves and their families. This chapter is concerned with the meanings and responsibilities that go with being a mother.

It begins by describing the place of motherhood in women's lives, noting how the expectation and experience of having children is the pivot around which the identity of many women turns. The central section of the chapter sets women's childcare role in the context of the domestic division of responsibility and labour within marriage, a division built around the principle that it is women who care for the home and the health of those who live there. The final section introduces a dimension of caring that can be easily obscured in accounts of motherhood that focus on feelings and relationships. It looks at how households organise their material resources to help (or hinder) women in meeting their caring responsibilities.

In contrast to Chapters 2 and 3, this chapter points to continuities and similarities in women's lives. It points to common patterns in the organisation of domestic life in Britain, both across time and between women.

4.2 Taking responsibility for children

The centrality of motherhood and caring for children runs as a thread of continuity between women. It is a dimension of gender that seems to transcend difference, framing the lives of women living in very different cultural and economic contexts. Women across these contexts describe how their future lives are closely tied into the expectation of becoming a mother (Beckett, 1986; Drury, 1991). They often see motherhood as central to their sense of self; the base on which a positive adult female identity is built.

Thus, Muslim women, like Sikh women, tend to define their futures in terms of becoming mothers (Afshar, 1989; Drury, 1991). White women often voice a similar commitment to motherhood (Oakley, 1979; Boulton 1983). Most of the White and African–Caribbean women in Phoenix's study, like respondents in other studies of young mothers, anticipated that having children would be the most fulfilling aspect of their lives and the experience that would confirm their adult status (Simms and Smith, 1986; Clark, 1989; Phoenix, 1991). Their feelings about motherhood are echoed in the accounts of mothers who adopt children and who care for children as stepmothers (Hughes. 1991). They are echoed, too, in the more limited evidence which records the experience of women coparenting children within a lesbian relationship (Hanscombe and Forster, 1981).

> I remember I just wanted to hold her all the time and not do anything else. Because of her disability, we had endless appointments with the physiotherapist, speech therapist, teacher, etc. and although I wanted to know what to do to help her, I sometimes resented all the time that it took. I just wanted to lie in bed with her, play and go for walks.
>
> I remember around our first Christmas feeling starry eyed and in love and not wanting to do anything else except be with her.[1]

> When I say I get depressed about things it's nowhere near as depressed as I would have been, I think, 'cos I've got him. He's like (pause) he makes everything worthwhile, all this hardship you go through, at least I've him. . . . before I had nothing 'n' I think I got more depressed about not having a baby . . . I've got this sense of well-being developed from having a kid, it's lovely, it's like having a love affair, you know, you've got all this contentment inside.[2]

The meanings and ideologies built around motherhood affect women who choose not to have children. They also affect women with fertility problems and health problems, which make pregnancy an unlikely prospect. Women confronting the possibility of childlessness are often more sharply aware of how much of their identity is wrapped up in becoming and being a mother (Woollett, 1991). In the accounts below, a woman undergoing treatment for infertility and a woman who is HIV positive talk about what motherhood means to them.

> One of the things I felt is that if you have children you become part of the human race. When I started to think about doing it, one of the complex things that made me want to, was that there would be a whole lot of things that I could share, that it would give me an enormous amount in common with most other people that otherwise you don't have.[3]

> When you're HIV positive and you're told you can't have any children or more of them, you feel terrible. It was another thing that made me feel different from all the other women I saw walking down the street and I definitely went through feeling an incredibly strong sense of being completely different from everyone else, and of being denied so much.[4]

A strong sense of being completely different comes through the accounts that mothers with disabled children have given of their lives (Hicks, 1988; Gregory, 1991). They describe the guilt and the grief and the loss of friends that often follow the birth of their baby and, with the passage of time, how they rebuild themselves and their social world on stronger and more secure foundations.

> We knew really, but I was heart broken, we knew when he was being tested; it was a shattering time that was; it was terrible but the thing is you have to keep telling yourself and make yourself try and accept it. The thing is I don't think you ever really do fully, fully accept it. I'm always waiting for one morning I'll get up and Colin will be alright, if I was dead honest about it, but really I know he won't be.[5]

> When I'd had the other two children all my friends came with cards and flowers. When I had Mark, nobody came. Nobody came to see me at home to talk about it. When Mark was two weeks old one very good friend saw us coming and crossed over the road. I crossed over and said to her, he's alive, we don't know how long we've got him, but for God's sake don't ignore me. I ended up having to say goodbye to fifteen to twenty friends. They don't know what to say or how to cope.[6]

As mothers with disabled children underline, being a mother means being continually and ultimately responsible for the welfare of your child. This sense of continual and ultimate responsibility runs through the accounts of motherhood provided by Black and White mothers, younger and older mothers, and by mothers in paid work, like those outside the labour market (Mayall, 1986; Brannen and Moss, 1988; Warrier, 1988; Phoenix, 1991). Disabled mothers often carry with them a particular determination, borne of childhood experiences in which they were segregated and overprotected, to help their children carve out independent lives for themselves. This theme is developed in the account below, where a disabled mother talks about the responsibility she feels for her disabled daughter.

> I was . . . frighteningly aware that the responsibility for giving this person a secure and happy childhood was entirely mine. There were people around to help with some of the practical tasks, but no one was going to share with me the actual responsibility for making it all work. This I felt to be awesome. I was probably more conscious than most mothers of the mistakes it is possible to make as a parent, as I had spent such a lot of time unpicking the tangle of my own childhood. . . . I think that my own early experience has, however, defined goals for me in my role as a parent. Despite all the work involved, I want her to grow up feeling that the world, and everything in it, is as much hers as anyone else's, and that she can be a powerful person who can affect her world as she chooses. I also want her to know that she is beautiful, touchable, loveable and not alone.[7]

Some mothers feel that their responsibilities for their children can be met by involving other people in the care of young children (Stone, 1983). In three-generational Muslim households, mothers have described a clear division of childcare responsibility among the women in the household. They have noted how it is usually the children's grandmother who does both the doting and the disciplining while they take on the domestic work associated with childcare (Afshar, 1989).

While others may be involved in the care of children, most mothers, at least when asked about their attitudes by researchers, emphasise that their children's needs are best met by them staying at home when their children are young. For example, in Phoenix's study of Black and White mothers under the age of 20, only one in twenty (5 per cent) were positively in favour of women with young children being in paid employment while four in ten (41 per cent) were against it (Phoenix, 1991). The lone mothers interviewed in the study by Bradshaw and Millar (1991) similarly identified their childcare responsibilities as the main reason for why they were not working. Studies focused on the experiences of Asian women have also noted how their childcare responsibilities were among the factors which propelled them into jobs in which they could earn money and look after their children at the same time (Afshar, 1989).

> I want to be a good mother first and foremost. What the children will remember is what their childhood was like. After all this is really the best thing that I could do for them to be with them and to get paid. What more do you expect? I could not leave them to other people to look after and my mother was getting too old and too tired, what with all the children she has had to raise, and all the worries. Her old age is really time for prayers and fasting and going to *haj*, not for baby minding.[8]

> I will stay at home and look after my kids at least until they start school. I think that children need their mothers. . . . I think that it's the woman who must look after the kids.[9]

Where mothers take on paid work, whether at home or outside it, the care and welfare of children usually remains their responsibility (Stone, 1983; Sharpe, 1984; Warrier, 1988; Afshar, 1989). In a study by Brannen and Moss on women returning to work after their first baby, both the mothers and their male partners felt it was the woman's responsibility to make arrangements for the care of the children, to pay for childcare and to ensure that the child's welfare did not suffer as a result of them going out to work (Brannen and Moss, 1988).

> It has been the bane of my life finding childcare and really the problem is still going on, like when he goes to school. When he was a baby trying to find a childminder was terrible, absolutely terrible – I used to spend my first three months in tears all the time – it was such a worry.[10]

Taking responsibility for the needs and care of young children involves many mothers in a day-long and life-long struggle to shield them against oppression and discrimination. Mothers caring for disabled children try to provide a supportive environment in which their children can build strong and resilient identities. Mothers caring for Black children and for children of mixed parentage work to construct a social world for them, at home, in their neighbourhood and at their school, which affirms their Black identity.

> . . . We live in a multi-racial area of London, where being Black is part of the norm. I am eternally grateful to our much maligned local authority for creating institutional support for schools such as Daniel's junior school which are prepared both to discuss and to outlaw racist behaviour. . . . Our part of London, and I mean the very local area, does not have noticeable levels of street racism. The atmosphere is a friendly one, and tension-free. Unfortunately, this has meant that I have gained little experience in dealing with these situations in an appropriate manner. I have little hesitancy in reacting to racial abuse when it is directed at others, but when confronted with racism directed against Daniel and myself, my breath has been taken away so entirely that I have dissolved into speechlessness.[11]

A woman's identity can leave her children vulnerable to pressures from which other children are protected. Jean Ellis, the author of the account given above, notes how racism shapes the reactions other people have to her and her son as a family unit in which she is White and he is Black (Ellis, 1992). Mothers have described the stigma their children face and fight when it is discovered that they live in a one-parent family and their mother is disabled or their mother is a lesbian (Goodman, 1980; MacPike, 1989; Morris, 1992a). Mothers who live on state benefits, either alone or with a partner, are also aware that their children can be given a hard time, both by adults and by children. As one father on benefit put it, 'the kids cop it because their dad's living off the state and all the rest of it, the taxpayers are paying your school dinners' (Cohen *et al.*, 1992, p.59).

> The people who worry me most are the children who go to school with my children. Because Julie and Liza are, naturally, not that strong yet, they can be hurt much more than I by a few nasty words. And because adults tend to talk behind one's back and not to one's face, I don't have to hear from my peers the kind of remarks my kids have to hear from theirs.
>
> Julie and I had another of those afternoons to ourselves

recently, and she told me that it bothers her when the kids at school make fun of gays.

'It just makes me so mad that I feel like sticking up for gays', she said. 'But if I did they'd think I was gay and make fun of me. So I just have to keep quiet about it'. . . .

So here is my biggest problem: I want to be a good mother. That means being honest with my children. It means instilling them with my own values and letting them be who they will be. It also means, while they are young, trying to shield them as much as possible from psychological harm.[12]

For women in these circumstances, the personal is unavoidably political. Caring for children means finding new and creative ways of living as a family, ways which counteract negative images and build positive self-identities.

When the children were very young, I was aware of being different from the many nuclear families around us – both friends and strangers. I would dread Bank Holidays and Sundays. We would go out and all I could see was nuclear families enjoying themselves. I felt our family was incomplete. Jessie has always been very attached to her father. She thoroughly enjoys the time she spends with him and misses him greatly. I did not want to add to her grief a feeling that we were inadequate as a family – a view reinforced by the media, my family, school, etc. In time, my feelings of 'incompleteness' went and today I feel this particular family is very complete indeed. With my increase of strength, I have noticed that Jessie no longer yearns for her father. She loves and misses him but feels secure.[13]

For women who experience the stigma of being different, there is the added pressure to prove that they are just as good as (if not better than) other mothers. This sense of having to make up a deficit runs through the accounts that young single women, lone mothers, stepmothers and disabled mothers have given of their lives (Clark, 1989; Hughes, 1991; Morris, 1992a).

We need not be supermums and dads, but as grumpy, confused, tired and scared as all other parents, without the fear that this will be interpreted as a sign that we are not coping. We also need to boast, to celebrate, to share our joys, insights, skills and discoveries with the world. For many disabled people, becoming a mother brings a fantastic feeling of creativity, belonging, womanhood, generosity and being part of the human race for the first time.[14]

4.3 Caring for families

Building a family that feels complete typically involves more than looking after children. It involves looking after the home and the well-being of all who live there. In most households, it is women who are the caretakers of the family, doing both the childcare and the domestic labour necessary to meet the needs of those who live in the household. In three-generational Asian households, the domestic labour, like childcare, is often shared among the women (and their daughters). However, as Brah (1992) notes in her study of women of Asian origin, with more members of the household to care for, a sharing of domestic labour does not necessarily mean less work for mothers.

The clustering of childcare responsibilities and domestic duties comes out clearly in studies based on couples living in nuclear, heterosexual households. The patterns recorded in Table 4.1 suggest that, in over 80 per cent of man–woman households, it is the woman who takes responsibility for childcare and for the care of the home (Witherspoon, 1988). It is women, too, who carry out most of the work involved in these duties: doing the household cleaning, the washing and the ironing, making the evening meal and looking after children when they are ill.

In one in five households, these responsibilities are carried out alongside the care of an adult or a disabled child who needs help with everyday tasks (Green, 1988). It is estimated that one in twenty households are providing 20 hours or more of informal care a week for someone who is disabled or sick. As Figure 4.1

Table 4.1 Patterns of responsibility and labour within marriage, Britain, 1987.

	%
Woman mainly responsible for:	
general domestic duties	82
general care of children	82
Woman mainly does:	
evening meal	77
household cleaning	72
washing and ironing	88
care of children when sick	67

Source: Jowell *et al.* (1988), Table 10.2 and text.

suggests, over half of Britain's carers live in households consisting of parents and children. Like childcare, informal care is a gendered responsibility. Two-thirds of those providing 20 or more hours of informal care a week are women and three in ten (29 per cent) have dependent children (Green, 1988). Qualitative studies record how caring for older relatives, like caring for children, is something that mothers, rather than fathers, do (Ungerson, 1987; Lewis and Meredith, 1988).

Women's employment status has a moderating influence on the patterns of domestic work mapped out in Table 4.1. Where women work full time, both overall responsibilities and individual tasks are more likely to be shared. In talking about their lives to researchers, women have described how their position as full-time workers makes it easier to renegotiate the divisions of domestic labour. Studies of Sikh women, for example, suggest that women's greater economic independence has given them the confidence to assert their need for more support at home (Bhachu, 1988; 1991).

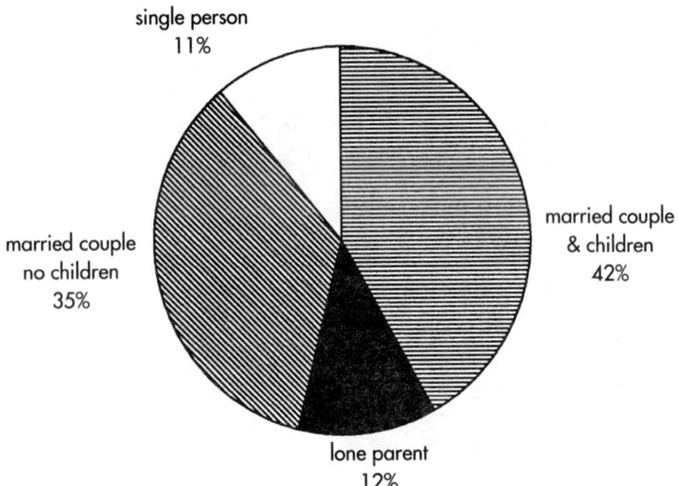

Figure 4.1 Carers devoting at least 20 hours a week to caring, by family type.

Note: Dependent children are persons under 16, or aged 16 but under 19 and in full-time education.
Source: Green (1988), derived from Table 2.18.

> I told my husband that he has to help me in the house because I can't manage with a full-time job. I too go out to work (kamai) just like him. I am just as tired when I come home as he is. I don't expect him to cook and clean more than me but I do expect him to listen to what I have to say. My take-home pay is almost as much as his, we couldn't manage without it.[15]

However, although the division of labour in households where women are in full-time paid work may be more equitable, it is not equal. The patterns described in Figure 4.2 suggest that, in the majority of these households, women remain responsible for domestic duties. They also typically carry out the domestic duties, making the evening meal, cleaning the home, and doing the washing and ironing. Among women in part-time work, gender equality appears to have made less headway. As Figure 4.2 records, the division of labour in households where women work part-time is little different from the patterns found in households in which women are not involved in paid work.

The domestic obligations of women in employment make for long working days and long working weeks. While spending less time on housework than women who are not in paid work, they

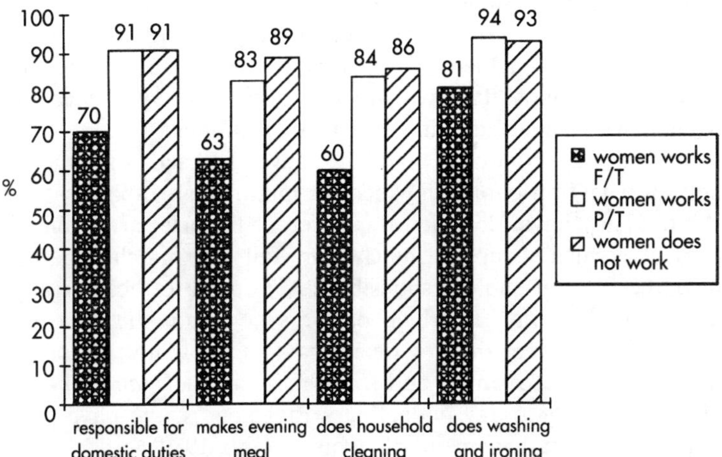

Figure 4.2 Domestic division of labour: responsibilities and tasks by women's employment status, Britain, 1987.

Source: Jowell *et al.* (1988), derived from Table 10.2.

are estimated to put in an average of 20 to 40 hours of domestic labour and childcare a week (Doyal, 1990). The heavy workload often offsets the potential health benefits which paid work can bring in terms of enhanced self-esteem, less isolation and a greater sense of autonomy. The health-enhancing effects of paid work can thus be limited by the difficulties women face in shedding domestic responsibilities.

Domestic responsibilities extend beyond the labour of housework and childcare. They include a resource management dimension, working to meet health needs within the income available.

4.4 Money for caring

In a minority of families, women play little part in the financial affairs of the household. In some three-generational Asian households, gender combines with kinship to vest authority over the control and management of resources in the senior women of the family and in the mother-in-law in particular (Bhachu, 1988; Afshar, 1989). In some nuclear families, too, women may have little experience of handling money and dealing with outside agencies for the payment of bills (Sadiq, 1991). But the evidence suggests that most families are organised in ways which vest women with significant financial responsibilities.

Studies of money in families have focused on nuclear, heterosexual households in which the majority of respondents are White. They have identified the different financial arrangements through which couples match (or fail to match) material resources to household responsibilities. Crucial to these arrangements are the ways in which partners negotiate the *control* of money (who makes the key decisions about how much money is made available to whom and for what) and the *management* of money (the day-to-day budgeting arrangements, the payment of bills and the management of debts) (Pahl, 1989).

Applying this typology, studies suggest that most heterosexual couples feel that money is organised in an egalitarian way, both jointly controlled and jointly managed (Witherspoon, 1988; Pahl, 1989).

> When we married we wanted to do everything together. We were both working then and it just carried on. It doesn't bother me not earning because I always have access to money. I don't feel dependent because I work quite hard for it: if it wasn't for the children I would be out at work anyway.[16]

However, the language of sharing and doing everything together can mask a reality in which control rests with one partner. Where this is the case, it is the man rather than the woman who is likely to make decisions about how money is shared out and who is responsible for different areas of expenditure. Male control over money tends to be reinforced by labour market position, with studies reporting that women exercise less control in homes where the man is the sole earner (L. Morris, 1990). It is mothers with young children who are most likely to live with men on whom they are financially dependent, leaving paid work in order to take on full-time caring (see Chapter 6). Male control of money, as women's accounts starkly record, is also woven into their experiences of violence in marriage. Women in violent relationships have described how their partner's control of money is one element in a relationship built on male dominance and female subordination (Dobash and Dobash, 1980; Evason, 1982; Pahl, 1985).

The management of money tends to have a rather different gender identity. It involves trying to implement decisions, working to meet financial responsibilities within the cash earmarked for them. For some women, this does not involve shopping and spending. None the less, for them, as for the majority of women who both shop and spend, resource management is an integral part of caring. Their health-keeping responsibilities involve housekeeping responsibilities: working to feed the family, heat the home and clothe the children within the money available. It is women, too, who work to keep up family standards and satisfy individual health needs when money is short (see Chapter 8).

The gendered patterns of control and management provide the context in which disagreements over money take place. In relationships where money is a cause of friction, women are more likely to voice concern about the financial control exercised by their partners, while noting that their partners are more likely to accuse them of financial mismanagement. Reflecting these tensions, women's lack of access to and control over money is a recurrent theme in their accounts of why their relationships broke down (Evason, 1980; Homer *et al.*, 1984).

> Sometimes we disagree about money, yes. He always says I spend too much. His hobby is fishing and do-it-yourself things and he'll just go out and buy the tools and I think, 'oh that money, what I could have done with that money'. So I will budget and go around the markets and that, and find the best buys and he'll just go to the best shop because it is convenient, so, yes, we disagree about money.

> Ronald didn't like me buying anything for the children. If I went out and bought them a pair of shoes and he wasn't with me, there was hell to pay when I got home. He just didn't like me spending money without his consent. If he wanted to go out and buy things that was different. He was very keen on photography and he bought a lot of photographic equipment. What things he wanted to buy was okay, but the basics and things I needed to get for the children, he thought were unreasonable.[17]

For mothers living outside marriage, issues of resource distribution can be resolved in different ways. For the majority of lone mothers, particularly those in their own accommodation, financial responsibility rests with them. In organising their financial affairs, lone mothers are able to combine the control and management of money into a single process. While two-parent households tend to develop complex control and management systems, lone mothers typically have one system in which they both control and manage the household income. The amount of money they receive, like the timing of its arrival, may be unpredictable, but once it has entered the home, it is usually theirs to organise and spend.

The issue of money looms large in the lives of most lone mothers. Becoming a lone mother often involves a movement out of a higher income household into a low-income household. It is therefore not surprising to find that most lone mothers report themselves to be considerably worse off as lone mothers. Bradshaw and Millar's study suggests that over half (54 per cent) of Britain's lone mothers feel themselves to be worse off than before they became lone mothers. However, a large minority (46 per cent) reported that they were no worse off or they were better off as lone mothers (Table 4.2). Over a quarter (27 per cent) described themselves as better off (Bradshaw and Millar, 1991). It is a finding echoed in other surveys. In a study of lone parents in Northern Ireland, three in ten (31 per cent) of the divorced mothers said they were better off living outside marriage than they had been within it (Evason, 1980). Where marital violence is a factor in becoming a lone mother, the proportion is appreciably higher. Two-thirds of those who took part in a survey of women in women's refuges reported that they were financially better off on their own (Binny *et al.*, 1985).

Male control of money emerges as a crucial factor in why some lone mothers feel better off. Their accounts suggest that they feel better off primarily because their control of household income has increased. Their access to a reliable source of income is more secure and, more particularly, they can have greater power over it. This suggests that being better off is a complex mixture of less money and more control. The complex mix is reflected in the reasons lone parents gave in Bradshaw and Millar's study for feeling better off as a lone parent. As Table 4.3 suggests, among those who registered an improvement in their financial circumstances, the main reasons related to the reliability of and control over their income. Over a quarter (28 per cent) said they felt better off because the money was now more regular and secure, while nearly a half (47 per cent) said it was because the money coming into the household was their own rather than their partner's (Bradshaw and Millar, 1991).

The patterns revealed in Tables 4.2 and 4.3 suggest that, for a

Table 4.2 Lone parents' comparisons of their financial situation, now and before they were a lone parent.

	%
A lot worse off now	38
A bit worse off now	16
The same now as before	19
A bit or much better off	27

Source: Bradshaw and Millar (1991), p.31.

Table 4.3 Reasons why lone mothers feel better off as a lone parent.

Main reason why they feel better off	%
Money was theirs, not their partners	47
Money more regular and secure	28
Fewer expenses	14
In paid employment	13

Source: Bradshaw and Millar (1991), p.31.

significant minority of women, lone motherhood involves less a movement into poverty and more a movement into a different kind of poverty. Instead of being poor within marriage, they are poor within the social security system.

> I'm much better off. Definitely. I know where I am now, because I get our money each week and I can control what I spend. Oh, he was earning more than I get but I was worse off then than I am now. At least I know where the money's being spent and it's not being spent. It might not last long but at least it's being put into provisions for the home.

> It's not easier or more difficult financially now. It's always been hard, now and when I was married, but for different reasons. I still owe money on the electricity and gas accounts. I only just have enough and I have to think, 'economise, economise!' all the time. But I feel better off because I have control of the money, even if I haven't got very much. He spent too much on silly things, like records and drink. Now I can budget for the bills.[18]

The accounts above suggest that, for some mothers, separation and lone parenthood are the best way of providing financial security for their children. The next chapter looks at how women organise the work of caring for children.

Notes

1. McKeith (1992), p.85–6.
2. Mother quoted in Fulop (1992), p.134.
3. Woman undergoing treatment for primary infertility quoted in Woollcett (1991), p.56.

4. Maggie in O'Sullivan and Thomson (eds) (1992), p.73.
5. Mother quoted in Gregory (1991), p.128.
6. Mother quoted in Hicks (1988), p.112.
7. Mason (1992), pp.116–17.
8. Mother quoted in Afshar (1989), p.223.
9. Young woman quoted in Drury (1991), p.397.
10. Mother quoted in Barry (1991), frontispiece.
11. Ellis (1992), pp.48–9.
12. Mansfield (1989), pp.92–3.
13. P. Murray (1992), pp.150–1.
14. Mason (1991), p.10.
15. Married woman quoted in Bhachu (1988), p.92.
16. Married mother quoted in Pahl (1989), p.72.
17. Married mother and lone mother quoted in Graham (1987a), p.63.
18. Two lone mothers quoted in Graham (1987a), p.65.

CHAPTER 5

CARING FOR CHILDREN

5.1 Introduction

Most of the 6.4 million mothers in Britain are living with children under the age of 11. Four in five (78 per cent) have one or more children in this age group. Nearly half (46 per cent) have at least one child under five. A relatively small proportion (22 per cent) only have children of secondary school age (Figure 5.1).

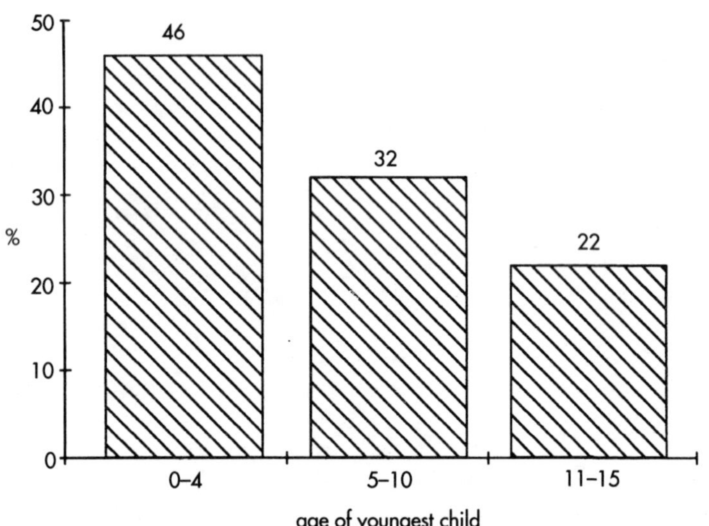

Figure 5.1 Women aged 16 to 59 living with children aged under 16 by age of youngest child, Britain, 1989.

Source: Employment Gazette (1990), p.930, derived from Table 6.

This chapter is concerned with women's domestic lives, looking, in particular, at the everyday routines which structure the lives of mothers with preschool children. The section below maps out these routines, describing the what, when and where of caring for young children. The subsequent section reviews the evidence which sheds light on the role that partners play in childcare, while the final section briefly reviews the help that comes from children and from women's networks beyond the home.

5.2 The what, when and where of childcare

As many mothers know, taking responsibility for children is hard work. The effort and energy that goes into their care is reflected in studies of budgeting time, which record how households with children clock up more hours of domestic labour than other households (Pahl, 1984). They also tend to be households in which there is least sharing of domestic labour. The gendered division of labour is at its sharpest in households with younger children, where most of Britain's mothers are to be found (see Figure 5.1).

In households with preschool children, the combined responsibilities of domestic labour and childcare makes for long working days for mothers – and often for disturbed nights. Fathers often play an important role, but one that centres on helping with rather than sharing responsibility for childcare. For example, the mothers with preschool children in Boulton's study all noted that, however much their husbands contributed, it was help with carrying out what was ultimately their responsibility (Boulton, 1983). In a study of parents caring for preschool children, women devoted an average of 374 minutes a week to basic childcare. The average among fathers was 47 minutes (Piachaud, 1984). In a more recent study of mothers with children under one year old, women spent a daily average of 14 hours on childcare and housework, while their fathers spent one hour a day in this way (Croghlan, 1991).

> I knew he was helping but it felt like it was ultimately my responsibility to look after her.[1]

> In my marriage, there was a very clear demarcation of roles. My husband earned the money, dealt with 'the world', and attended to all household maintenance. I had responsibility for everything else – primarily child care. Child care and the constraints of parenting were an optional extra for him. My life was fragmented by attending to others, his could follow an uninterrupted flow.[2]

Mothers' domestic lives are marked out not only by their long hours of domestic labour. The 'what' of their domestic lives, like the 'where' and 'when' of childcare, build a distinctive daily routine (Cullen, 1979). The subsections below look at the dimensions of what, where and when in turn.

(*i*) *The what of mothers' lives*

The what of mothers' lives consists primarily of activities that they perceive to be part of their daily routine. They are activities that tend to be carried out in the same way everyday. The routine nature of domestic life was vividly recorded by mothers who took part in a study which I conducted in the mid-1980s. The study included women with preschool children living in a variety of circumstances (as lone mothers and as married/cohabiting mothers, for example), as well as with a diversity of class, cultural and ethnic backgrounds (Graham, 1986). The 105 mothers in the study were asked to complete a 24-hour diary of their activities. They recorded over 80 per cent of their activities as routine, as part of the normal pattern of their lives. These routine activities involved getting children up, washing, feeding and dressing them, taking older children to school and playgroup (escort journeys), watching over and supervising younger children, and preparing the evening meal for their partners. These routines, in turn, were structured by the timetable of other people's needs: by meal times and sleep times, by school times and their partners' hours of work. Living within the timetable of other people's needs can mean routines of waiting rather than doing. The domestic world, as Carolyn Steedman puts it, is 'full of women waiting' (Steedman, 1986, p.22).

> You're on the go from seven in the morning and you're on call more or less all night, every night, whereas you're not when you're working. Your boss isn't going to ring you up at eleven o'clock at

> night and say come and take a letter. Whereas if the baby cries, you can't say I've finished for the day, tough luck.

> I went to bed about half past twelve, got up at seven. I got up three times in the night . . . [then] I fed him about a quarter to nine. Fed him, washed my hair, I had a couple of biscuits. I fed him and then I dashed down to the shops . . . as soon as we came back it was time to feed him again.[3]

The mothers in the study recorded how other caring-related routines were fitted into the dominant time structures of children and partners. Their diaries described how they shopped and cooked, washed and ironed, cleaned and cleared away in the spaces of the day when they were not directly attending to the needs of children and partners. These snatches of time were also claimed for another set of routines which were more related to mothers' own needs. These were the self-directed routines, principally of the coffee and tea variety, where mothers took a brief break from housework and childcare. Such breaks often had a special significance, symbolic and material, for lone mothers who otherwise could find themselves with little or no adult time. The interweaving of these different kinds of routine is illustrated in the half-day diaries of two mothers with preschool children, one married mother and one lone mother, reproduced in Tables 5.1 and 5.2.

For some mothers, time to themselves is further limited by the special needs of their children. Caring for a disabled child typically means that more time and energy is invested in childcare tasks such as lifting, carrying, feeding and dressing. Caring can also involve a closer and more constant emotional involvement. Mothers may spend more time designing activities for a child who may be easily bored and fractious, and providing supervision for a child who is not safe if left alone (Glendinning, 1983; Read, 1991). Such attention and supervision can continue into the night, with disturbed sleep being part of the routine of motherhood, part of the normal pattern of daily (or rather nightly) life. Whereas other mothers may look to the support of neighbours and friends to help them through, women with disabled children can find themselves isolated within their local communities. Studies have recorded how they often live outside the informal networks that keep other mothers going (Read, 1991). Faced

Table 5.1 A mother's half-day diary: mother living with a male partner and two children, aged 6 and 4.

			Main activity	
Time	Main activity	Other activity	Routine? (Y/N)	Others there?
6.15	Get up, make morning drinks	Wake up husband	Y	No-one
6.35	Went back to bed – unusual, but feeling tired	Children playing	N	2 children
7.40	Got up, saw husband off	Got washed, dressed, let cat out	Y	No-one
8.00	Children to bathroom	Filling in diary	Y	2 children
8.10	Chase children	Tidy bedrooms	Y	2 children
8.15	Find them clothes to wear	Sort out dirty linen	Y	2 children
8.25	Chase older son/ washing up	Redress younger child	Y	2 children
8.30	Breakfast	Chase older son, help daughter with shoes, feed cat	Y	2 children
8.40	Get ready for school	Answer son's countless questions	Y	2 children
8.45	Clear breakfast table	Check children	Y	2 children
8.55	Out the door!	Hurrying children on	Y	2 children
9.00	Leave son at school		Y	2 children
9.05	Take daughter to playgroup		Y	1 child
9.30	Leave daughter at playgroup	Talk to play-group leader – daughter becoming unsettled	Y	1 child

Table 5.1 *continued*

9.35	Family planning appointment		N	Doctors, nurses, patients
11.00	Arrive back home		N	No-one
11.05	Housework	Coffee	Y	No-one
11.45	Collect daughter from playgroup	Talk to play-group leader – to see if she is more settled	Y	1 child
12.00	Collect son from school	Talk to children	Y	2 children
12.20	Prepare lunch	Persuade children to sit down	Y	2 children

Source: Graham (1985), p.199.

Table 5.2 A mother's half-day diary: lone mother with two children, aged 6 and 3.

			Main activity	
Time	Main activity	Other activity	Routine? (Y/N)	Others there?
12.15	Prepare lunch	Supervising child	Y	Child
12.30	Eat	Supervising child	Y	Child
1.00	Wash up	Supervising child	Y	Child
1.30	Cup of coffee and a cigarette	Supervising child	Y	Child
2.00	2 friends call, make coffee	Playing with children	N	Child
3.00	Collect older child from school		Y	Children
3.15	Get drinks for children	Talking to children	Y	Children
4.00	Start preparing dinner	Talking to children	Y	Children

Table 5.2 *continued*

Time	Main activity	Other activity	Main activity Routine? (Y/N)	Others there?
4.15	Washing up	Supervising children	Y	Children
4.30	Put toys away with children		Y	Children
4.45	Set table	Supervising children	Y	Children
5.00	Get washing in		Y	Children
5.15	Eat dinner	Supervising children	Y	Children
5.45	Washing up	Supervising children	Y	Children
6.00	Sit down, have cigarette	Supervising children	Y	Children
6.10	Helped older child with homework	Supervising child	Y	Children
6.30	Get children ready for bed		Y	Children
6.45	Give children milk		Y	Children
6.50	Watched TV with children		Y	Children
7.00	Put children to bed		Y	Children
7.30	Make coffee		Y	No-one
7.35	Watched TV with 2 friends		Y	Friends
9.00	Make packed lunch for older child		Y	No-one
9.15	Washed up		Y	No-one
9.45	Had a bath		Y	No-one
10.15	Went to bed		Y	No-one
10.30	See to older child		N	No-one
10.45	Back to bed		N	No-one

Source: Graham (1985), p.197.

with the insensitive behaviour of others, mothers can also withdraw from contact with friends in an attempt to protect themselves and their children from hurt.

> First of all, in the morning, Andrew's got to be got up and dressed and fed and toileted, and you know he's got to be *held* on the toilet – you can't leave him. It's a couple of hours, really. And you can't do anything else while you are feeding him. If you turn round, it's spat out. It's a couple of hours getting him ready for school. And then when he comes home at half past three, your time is devoted to him. Someone has to be there. And when he goes to bed, you're constantly turning him. He has to be turned so many times before he goes to sleep. And he can be sick three times a night.[4]

Caring responsibilities can extend beyond those that mothers have for their children. There may be adult members of the household who also find it difficult to live independently. The few studies which have recorded the experiences of mothers who are also informal carers point to the way in which women struggle to keep family life as undisturbed as possible for partners and children. Mothers work hard to keep up standards in the face of an increasing volume of domestic work and personal care (Lewis and Meredith, 1988).

> You feel all the responsibility is yours. They're only doing it to help you but the whole responsibility is mine. It was a big burden, a very big burden . . . It was a struggle. It was all so new, so sudden. It just took all the time, there was nothing else I could do. I just managed to do the washing – bung it in the machine. There were shirts piling up . . .[5]

(ii) The when of mothers' lives

It is not only the what of mothers' lives that distinguishes their lifestyles from those of their partners. The when of their lives, too, tends to have a distinctive tempo. In one study of the paid and unpaid work of married couples, men's work activities were typically concentrated between 7.00 a.m. and 6.00 p.m., peaking at 10.00 a.m. and 3.00 p.m. (Cullen, 1979). The work patterns of their wives were more complex. Like their husbands, the housewives rose early and were busiest during the morning. As other surveys suggest, mornings are the time for housework and laundry; they are also times for shopping and escort journeys. Among the women in the study, the domestic peak fell gradually in the afternoon, but rose sharply again in the late afternoon and early evening. By 7.30 p.m., one-third of the women in employment and one-third of the women who worked only for their families were still at work in their homes (Cullen, 1979).

Early evenings is when the timetables of children and partners converge. In the space of a few hours in the early evening, cooking, eating, washing up, bathtimes and bedtimes all have to be completed – at a time when mothers have been working for upwards of ten hours. Not surprisingly, the early evening is often identified as a crisis time by mothers.

> I think looking after children is the hardest job going and the one where you get the least preparation and training for. To be quite honest, that's how I feel. Very, very demanding in time, energy, affection and it's not a job you've got from nine in the morning till five at night. It's 24 hours a day, especially as my son has only just started going through the night and he's four and a half. Very demanding on all fronts. Demanding 24 hours of attention is a bit much and I think you need – well I need – a time without them to regain a little bit of sanity.[6]

(iii) The where of mothers' lives

Turning from the when to the where of mothers' lives, studies have highlighted their homecentredness. For some women, homecentredness may reflect religious and cultural beliefs. Among practising Muslims, for example, women may develop patterns of interaction and visiting which focus on the home and within the extended family (Currer, 1991). Homecentredness does not only stem from religious values, however. The organisation of childcare within families means that the majority of mothers with preschool children live their lives in and around the home.

The homecentredness of mothers' lives came out clearly in the diary-based study introduced earlier in the section. The diaries suggested that the mothers spent an average of 75 per cent of their day in the house. A third of their day was spent in the kitchen. The main reasons for leaving the home were shopping and visiting relatives and friends. These activities, like the home-based routines, were carried out with their children. As other studies have confirmed, most mothers live their lives with, as well as for, their children (Mayall, 1986). In a survey of 900 mothers with babies six months' old, 96 per cent were with their baby for most of the day. Only the small minority in paid work had time away on a regular basis from their children (Graham, 1992a).

> I think it's so all-consuming. I think you do love them so much, you do love them very much indeed. And I think again if it's a bad day outside, or she's not very well and you're indoors all the time, it does get on top of you because you feel, you know, I should be able to cope with all this and of course sometimes you can't.

> Sometimes I feel like this is a prison. I don't miss work, I miss the company of work. Sometimes it can be a bit boring with just children every day but then, other times I quite enjoy being on my own with them. But just now and again it gets on top of you. You just feel like knocking down the walls, getting rid of housework and carpets.[7]

Spending time at home may reflect the fact that mothers are, as studies put it, 'communication and transport-deprived' (Pearson *et al.*, 1992, p.10). Households on a low income and with a head of household who is unemployed or in an unskilled manual job are less likely to have a telephone than those that are better-off with an employed head of household and with a professional job (Office of Population Censuses and Surveys, 1991a). Car ownership displays a similar class gradient. Less than six in ten (59 per cent) households with an unemployed or unskilled manual head have a car or van. Among professional households, the proportion is 95 per cent. Based on household-ownership, these statistics provide an unreliable guide to women's access to private transport.

Women are less likely than men to have driving licences. The family car, too, tends to travel with the man to work, leaving women dependent on other means of transport. The relative 'transport deprivation' of women came across clearly in a recent study of working-class mothers. Over 60 per cent lived in households with a car or van. However, only a third (33 per cent) of the mothers had access to the car on weekdays (Graham, 1992a). As other studies confirm, while men travel by car, women walk (Beuret, 1991).

> If I want to go somewhere, I have to wait for him to come home or start walking. But both of us driving would be expensive. I don't really think we could afford it. I go to the local shops if I haven't got time to go to the shopping centre but if I've plenty of time, I walk to the shopping centre. If the market's on, I'd definitely walk in because it's a lot cheaper.

> To cart a baby around on the bus would kill me, with pushchairs and shopping and things like that. So Dave (husband) does the big shop. He goes twice a week on the bus to the shopping centre. I never use the buses. I walk everywhere.[8]

For mothers who live home-based lives, their quality of life is more closely linked to the physical environment of home and neighbourhood than it is for people who spend much of their time away from home and without children. The physical environment is frequently not a health-promoting one. Poor housing conditions often go along with busy roads and lack of safe playspace. In addition to these hazards, many mothers identify the presence of dogs as a source of danger to their children. A significant minority of mothers report that they, too, do not feel safe on the streets (Sexty, 1990; Graham, 1992a). The accounts of Black mothers also highlight how they restrict their children's freedom to play out because of racist attacks in the streets, in the local park – and in their own backyards (Currer, 1991).

> . . . around here there doesn't seem to be too much to do. . . . I try to get him out every day; now he's walking he wants to walk everywhere, and he can't. It's such a busy area, main roads, I can't let him. . . . So normally we take a walk . . . just looking at the shops. I try to take him places where there's a lot of colour and a lot of light. He's television mad at the moment, but that's all he ever sees is television.[9]

The physical environment of the home and neighbourhood can be a particularly important issue for mothers in poor health or whose mobility is restricted. As one disabled mother observed of her daughter's lifestyle, 'most of Rosa's activities occur in places which are inaccessible to me. The drama class she goes to, the music club, most of her friends' houses – all these are places where I cannot enter' (Morris, 1992b, p.134).

> I believe that the experience of disabled parents is profoundly relevant to all parents and to those who work with them. Disabled parents face the difficulties which all parents face, but the effects are frequently exacerbated by the presence of physical impairments. I am talking here about such things as exhaustion, isolation, inappropriate housing, juggling limited resources, the unwelcoming attitudes of places such as shops and restaurants and the inaccessibility of many public buildings. At the same time, because disabled parents are amongst those most harshly affected by the constraints and under-resourcing of parents in our society, we are also amongst those who are furthest along the road to finding solutions. This is one of the reasons why our experience is worth looking at.[10]

As mothers' accounts remind us, there are divergent as well as common patterns in the what, when and where of their domestic lives. Mothers differ in the kinds of responsibilities they face and the context in which they face them. They differ, too, in the support they get from others in meeting their responsibilities. It is the question of help in the home that is explored in the final two sections of this chapter.

5.3 Help from partners

Many mothers receive little support from others in shouldering either the responsibility or the labour of childcare. Lone mothers, for example, often have little time away from their children and little help from others. As Table 5.2 indicates, nearly all their waking hours may be spent with their children.

> It feels alright – I'm quite happy. It's as difficult as I thought. I think it's worse than I thought because I didn't think kids could be so much of a handful as he is. I've looked after a lot in the past and none of them has been like him. People say isn't he sweet and lovely but I say no, you have him for a week – he's something different. It would be nice to say, 'I've had enough, you have him for ten minutes while I go and soak in the bath'. If I want a bath, he's got to go with me.[11]

Women living with others have greater opportunities to share, if only in part, the emotional and physical responsibility of caring for children. For mothers with young children, male partners are often the primary source of emotional as well as financial support. At a time when women are heavily dependent, both emotionally and economically, on their partners, they can place a relatively low premium on his active involvement in childcare and housework (Boulton, 1983; Croghlan, 1991). Recognising his vital contribution, women often express little dissatisfaction with a domestic division of labour that leaves them with both the responsibility and the work of caring.

> Martin works very hard, that's *his* work for the family. I run the home so he *can* work hard. There is too much emphasis these days on what a father's *got* to do. He hasn't *got* to do anything. Not all fathers want to or can get involved, but you're made to feel guilty if your husband is not like the ideal dad.

> He's never here when she gets up, so really he is best playing with her. He doesn't have time for shopping or housework. He would if he were here. He works six days a week. He's one of those, you know, who the only time he rests is in the evening when he gets home and just conks out. He can play with her while he's sitting resting.[12]

In relationships where the threat of violence is a constant undercurrent, women can be particularly reluctant to challenge the domestic division of labour. Women report how violent attacks often centre around sexual jealousy and domestic work, set off by what are taken to be challenges to their partner's authority. As Dobash and Dobash (1980) note, male expectations concerning women's domestic role and, particularly, the preparation and serving of food, are commonly the context for the first violent attack (p.95). In such circumstances, any domestic help from partners may be experienced as wholly negative and mothers may welcome the fact that their partners are unwilling to take more responsibility for childcare and housework (Croghlan, 1991).

Where male partners take on more than financial and emotional support, the evidence suggests that they occupy a particular niche in the organisation of care. As noted earlier, they are more likely to adopt the role of assistant than that of equal partner (Brannen and Moss, 1988). As helpers, men gravitate more to childcare than to housework and figure less strongly in the more mundane and routine areas of household work (Brannen and Moss, 1988; Croghlan, 1991). Thus, on the housework side, they typically prefer, and are more involved in, shopping, cooking and clearing away. They are less likely to take on washing up, washing clothes and ironing. Similarly, in relation to childcare, partners are more involved in child-focused activities like bathing, playing and putting to bed. They do less in the way of nappy-changing, feeding and getting up in the night to attend to children.

> He doesn't help as much as I would like. He might take Joanna out if he went over to the shops or keep an eye on her if I went out but he doesn't do things like giving her a bath or giving her her tea or getting her ready for bed or anything like that. My husband thinks a woman's place is in the home and a woman must do what a woman must do. The husband's job is to bring in the bread, which he's not doing now he's unemployed! A lot of my friends' husbands do help out. They think nothing of bathing the children or putting the hoover around. As long as he has his dinner on the table and clean clothes for his back and he can do what he wants when he wants, he's alright.[13]

5.4 Help from others

While there is an increasing interest in the role of fathers, much less attention has been given by researchers to the contribution made by children to the domestic economy. It is, however, a contribution that women have highlighted in their accounts of their lives. As with partners, it is emotional support that women tend to emphasise, with their relationships with children represented in ways which underline how much love children give as well as receive. The importance of children as a source of emotional support shines through particularly strongly in the accounts of mothers who find their personal identities – as Black, as disabled, as lesbian, as one-parent, as poor or as all of these – leave them vulnerable to self-doubt and discrimination from others (Ross, 1988; MacPike, 1989; Morris, 1989; 1992a).

> My tiredness and depression sometimes erupted into violence,

> swiftly followed by agonising guilt. It was a guilt compounded by the knowledge that I had little money, I was a white mother of a black child in a racist society and, above all, I had chosen to have her. I could only blame myself as I got more scared of how this dangerous and difficult world could damage my child. It was I who thought it possible and had obstinately refused to listen to warnings. . . .
>
> Somehow things changed and I have no idea why or even exactly when. As Ella learnt to walk, to understand more, to play with other children, I rediscovered a pride and delight in being part of her growing. . . . Whatever the cause, I felt her pulling me back from my worst fears. It was as if she was saying, through her energetic presence, don't waste time complaining about life, get on and live it.[14]

Alongside mothers' autobiographical records are a handful of studies which have highlighted the material contribution that children make to the household. These studies have noted both the extent of paid child labour in Britain and the significant unpaid input that many children make to the running of the home (Hobbs *et al.*, 1992). The limited evidence suggests that children's domestic contribution begins by their taking responsibility for themselves (L. Morris, 1990). Self-maintenance is clearly a significant but largely unrecorded dimension of family life, with children preparing their meals, tidying their rooms and looking after themselves when in the home alone. Studies of Muslim families have recorded how young children are involved in wider household activities, gaining first-hand experience by helping to look after younger siblings and by taking part in housework (Currer, 1991). In White households, children appear to be older before they start to make a direct contribution to domestic labour (L. Morris, 1990).

A recent study used essays on 'What I do when I am not at school' to collect information on the domestic labour of 700 young people aged 11 to 16 (Morrow, 1992). Their domestic tasks included housework (washing up, ironing, tidying up, etc.), childcare (caring and babysitting for siblings or cousins), shopping and outdoor household tasks, such as car-washing and lawn-mowing. The study suggested that four in ten young people were involved in domestic activities, with girls more likely to help than boys. Thus, less than a third of the boys but over half of the girls were involved in domestic labour. Other studies have underlined how this gender division is part of the socialisation of daughters into their female role. In Afshar's study of three-generational Muslim households, mothers noted how they trained their daughters in housework, cooking, sewing and mending, with daughters assigned a clear role in the domestic economy. Thus, the oldest daughter was often charged with the housework, while the second did the cooking and the third daughter was the one who was educated beyond 16 (Afshar, 1989).

Gender relations are affirmed by the receiving as well as the giving of care, with children's labour constructed as 'helping mum'. In Morrow's study, the young people nearly always described how they helped their mothers with household chores. There were only a few instances of 'helping Dad'. The young people in the study identified parental employment as a major factor shaping their involvement in domestic labour, contributing to the housework, cooking and childcare 'because my mum works'. Children also appear to do more for their mothers in households where mothers are bringing them up on their own.

> I do help my mum with the housework. I polish, change the sheets, hoover and clean the bathroom every Saturday. And when we are on half-term or holidays, I clean the house every day for my mum. I wash up every night and sometimes cook the meal. (15-year-old girl)

> I do the washing up every day and I always go round the shop for my mum, my mum gives me £3.00 pocket money. Sometimes mum gives me extra money if I do shopping for her. Sometimes I get rid of spiders for my mum. I put oil in the car and water in the radiator for my mum every three weeks. I make tea for my mum in the morning. As I want to be a chef, I sometimes cook dinner for my mum and my brother. (12-year-old boy)

> I help a lot at home because my mum and dad are at work until about half past six, so when I get home I usually tidy the kitchen and living room, and then cook dinner for mum and dad and then I sit down and do my homework until they get home. (12-year-old girl)[15]

It is not only partners and children who play an important role in helping women with their domestic responsibilities. Other relatives within the home also make an important contribution.

The support provided by other household members – and their mothers in particular – comes across particularly clearly in the accounts that young women have given of caring for children (Clark, 1989; Phoenix, 1991). The relatives and friends who make up women's networks beyond the home, too, provide resources which lift some of the burdens off women with young children. These networks can provide substitute care and access to transport on a routine basis, enabling mothers to go shopping without their children and without time-consuming journeys by foot or public transport. The role of social networks has been highlighted, particularly, in relation to access to health services, where resources held by relatives and friends, such as substitute care, a telephone or a car, are carefully 'saved up' by mothers to be used for hospital appointments and emergencies (Pearson *et al.*, 1992).

Within women's social networks, it is relatives who are usually the most reliable and frequent source of substitute care and transport. Their importance has been highlighted in studies of mothers caring for non-disabled children and, particularly, for disabled children (Meltzer *et al.*, 1989). Women often identify their mothers from among kin as the most important source of help from outside the household. Loans of money and gifts of food and clothes provided by their mothers underwrite the budgeting strategies of many women struggling to make ends meet (see Chapters 7 and 8). Although providing important material resources, however, it is the emotional and social support of families that women with young children value most.

> She (mother) is marvellous with them. If I need a babysitter, she'll come up if she can. She works, but if she's got a week off, she'd have them. She's my best friend really. It sounds old-fashioned but she is. You can say anything to your mum! I can have a good moan at her and she won't think anything the worse of you. I'd like to see more of her but I can't because of not being able to afford to get down and she can't afford to get up here.[16]

> At first I didn't react at all: I didn't know she had Down's syndrome until she was six weeks old; I couldn't see it, I suppose I could say I didn't believe it. I just didn't acknowledge it for a few weeks. . . . My mother was absolutely devastated, she was. She told me later that she cried for three years. But having said that, she's been so good to me. After I had Nina, I've become so close

> to her. . . . My mum is absolutely fantastic: she writes letters to Nina, Nina is very special to her. I think they're very, very close.[17]

Like other sources of help, not all mothers have access to family networks. Parents may not live in Britain. They may have died or split up while other relatives may have moved away. The lives of women, too, may change in ways that fracture their family networks. A separation or divorce may tear family ties; women may be rehoused following the birth of their children or their financial circumstances may change in ways which make it hard to afford public transport and impossible to run a car or pay for a telephone. While shortage of money can make it difficult to keep in contact with family and friends, these social networks provide a vital source of childcare for mothers looking for paid work to increase their family's income. The patterns of women's paid work are the focus of the next chapter.

> It was my mother I felt close to, if anybody, when she was alive. There's no one really. It used to be my mum, she used to get all my troubles but I don't tell anyone anything now. More or less keep it to myself, and that's why you get depressed because you've got no one to talk to.

> My parents are split up. My mother lives in Manchester, and I see her a few times a year. She'll knit jumpers for my daughter and get her things in jumble sales. I've lost contact with my father. Mike's parents are split up too. His father lives in Wolverton and I see him once a week. But he works and is very busy. If we needed money, he'd help out but not really in any other way. His mother has moved away, I've only met his mother once.[18]

Notes

1. Mother quoted in Croghlan (1991), p.229.
2. Hope (1992), pp. 65–6.
3. Mother quoted in A. Oakley (1979), pp.241, 239.
4. Mother of a 15-year-old severely disabled son quoted in Baldwin (1985), p.78.
5. Women caring for children and their disabled mothers quoted in Lewis and Meredith (1988), p.79.
6. Married mother, unpublished data from Graham (1985).

7. Two mothers living with partners, Graham, unpublished data.
8. Two mothers living with partners, Graham, unpublished data.
9. Lone mother quoted in Miller (1990), p.40.
10. Wates (1991), pp.9–10.
11. Lone mother quoted in Clark (1989), p.29.
12. Two married mothers quoted in Graham (1985), pp.171–2.
13. Married mother quoted in Graham (1985), p.172.
14. Phillips (1992), pp.157–8.
15. Young people quoted in Morrow (1992), pp.11, 15 and 18.
16. Mother quoted in Graham (1985), p.160.
17. Mother quoted in Hicks (1988), pp.116–18.
18. Two mothers living with partners quoted in Graham (1985), p.166.

CHAPTER 6

WORKING FOR PAY

6.1 Introduction

The last chapter pointed to the differential impact of children on women and men. It is mothers rather than fathers whose domestic lives are built around the needs and welfare of children. This chapter looks at the position of mothers in the labour market. Here, too, the evidence points to the difference that gender makes. It suggests that the arrival of children heralds changes in women's working lives, changes from which most men are protected. Women typically give up paid work when they become mothers, often taking on lower paid and less secure part-time jobs when they return to the labour market as their children get older.

Lone mothers often find their employment options are particularly restricted. Their patterns of employment, like those of married and cohabiting women, are being shaped by wider changes in women's employment. These changes, in turn, are part of a restructuring of the British economy, a process of change which has gained momentum through the 1980s and 1990s.

The section below looks at the trends in women's employment in the context of these wider economic changes. The subsequent section is concerned with how women view their decisions about paid work. The chapter then reviews the evidence on the patterns of paid work among mothers before examining, in the final section, the patterns and problems of paid work for lone mothers.

6.2 Trends in women's employment

In the 1940s and 1950s, women's traditional pathways through marriage and motherhood (outlined in Chapter 2) were matched by a traditional approach to paid work. Forty years ago most women got married in their early twenties and gave up work. Today, most married women are in paid employment (Office of Population Censuses and Surveys, 1991a).

Within this upward trend, there are marked differences between women in their access to employment. Disabled women face particular disadvantages, both in finding work and in finding work commensurate with their skills and qualifications (Lonsdale, 1990). The OPCS surveys of disability suggest that less than three in ten (29 per cent) disabled women of working age are in paid work: among women as a whole in Britain, two-thirds (66 per cent) are in full-time or part-time work (Martin *et al.*, 1989; *Employment Gazette*, 1990).

'Race' is also structured into women's employment experiences. The search for secure employment brought many African–Caribbean women to Britain where they joined the increasing number of White women entering the labour market (Phizacklea, 1982). Over seven in ten African–Caribbean and White women of working age are economically active (in paid employment or unemployed) (*Employment Gazette*, 1991). For many Asian women coming to Britain from the Indian subcontinent, paid work represented a break with past traditions. It brought with it their first experience of paid employment (Wilson, 1978). Today, six in ten women identified as Indian in the Labour Force Survey are economically active (*Employment Gazette*, 1991). For women from Bangladesh and Pakistan, who are among the most recently arrived groups in Britain, economic activity rates are considerably lower. Two in ten Bangladeshi and Pakistani women of working age are in employment or looking for work (*Employment Gazette*, 1991). Among the factors which explain their lower rates of economic activity is the greater involvement of Bangladeshi and Pakistani women in childcare. As noted in Chapter 2, a high proportion of women in these groups are in households with children (see Figure 2.3). Further, those seeking to combine the care of their children with paid work have had to do so in the face of rising unemployment. However, the under-recording of homeworking/homesewing means that economic activity rates are likely to be higher among women whose ethnic identity is recorded as Bangladeshi and Pakistani than official data suggest (Bhachu, 1991).

A significant proportion of women in the labour market work part time. Labour Force Survey data relating to White, Indian and West Indian women indicate that part-time work is more common among White women. Full-time work is a more dominant pattern among Black women (*Employment Gazette*, 1991). Asian and African–Caribbean women are also more likely to work shifts, and work night shifts, than White women (Oppenheim, 1990).

The growth of women's employment has coincided with two particular trends: an increase in unemployment and a shift towards low paid, part-time work in the service sector of the economy. Firstly, women's employment increased through the 1960s, 1970s and 1980s at a time when the levels of full-time male employment were falling. The increase in unemployment hit those in marginal positions in the labour market. It was, and is, concentrated among young people and people in semi-skilled and unskilled manual occupations (Heady and Smyth, 1989). The evidence also suggests that among parents with dependent children, it is parents in the younger age groups and parents with three or more children who are most likely to be unemployed.

The age structure of Black communities means that Asian and African–Caribbean families have been hit particularly hard by the rise in youth unemployment and by the patterns of unemployment among parents. Black workers also face the additional disadvantages of a labour market structured around 'race' inequalities. The cumulative impact of these disadvantages is a rate of Black unemployment which is consistently higher than the White unemployment rate, with the difference narrowing in times of economic boom and widening in times of recession (Brown, 1990).

The upward trend in women's employment has coincided, secondly, with a decline in employment in the manufacturing industries and an expansion of the service sector. The number of people employed in the manufacturing sector (in textiles, engineering, shipbuilding, steel and metal manufacture, etc.) fell by over a third in the 1970s and 1980s, while the number of employees in the service sector rose by a third over the same period (Central Statistical Office, 1992). Nearly 70 per cent of those in paid work now work in the service industries.

The growth of service-sector employment has been fuelled by the development of what is known, somewhat euphemistically, as 'flexible work'. Flexible types of work include part-time work, self-employment, temporary or seasonal work, and homeworking. Within these types of flexible working, it is part-time work (which is often temporary and home-based) which represents the largest category (Huws *et al.*, 1989). Part-time work is an increasingly common type of work and represents a significant part of the expansion of service-sector employment. In the second half of the 1980s, the number of full-time employees grew by 6 per cent while the number of part-time workers increased by 14 per cent. Today, one in five people in paid employment works part time (Office of Population Censuses and Surveys, 1991b).

The increase in women's employment is closely meshed into the growth of flexible working and service-sector employment. It is estimated that over half of all women in employment are part of the flexible labour force and four in five (81 per cent) work in the service industries (Lewis and Bowlby, 1989; *Employment Gazette*, 1990). Low pay is also associated with women's work, particularly for those in manual occupations and part-time work. Eight in ten women in full-time manual work are low paid; among those in part-time manual work, the proportion is nine in ten (*New Review*, 1991a; b). Homeworking, too, is a highly gendered form of flexible working. It is estimated that over 70 per cent of homeworkers are women (Hakim, 1987). Low-paid, unskilled employment typically gives women little control over their work which, as a result, is often monotonous and uncreative. Combined with the demands of caring, it can put a strain on women's emotional and physical health (Doyal, 1990).

> Sometimes I think I could throw all this work out of the window. Sometimes it gets on top of you. I just feel I want to pack it all in. I want to get miles away. I just can't go on any more. I don't want to go home and start getting the tea, but I do. It sometimes comes on during the day, when I'm working or at home. And then I feel I would like to go to the doctor and be able to have a few days off, just to stop worrying.[1]

The data reviewed in this section give a sense of what women do in the labour market. However, they reveal little about why they do it. This issue is explored in the next section.

6.3 Why women work

There are three clusters of reasons why women work. Firstly, women have emphasised the social relations of paid work. Paid work can be a source of self-esteem. By providing social contact and companionship, it can also help to break the isolation of women's domestic lives.

> I wouldn't like the idea of working full-time but getting out for a couple of hours, it gives me a break, and at least I've got some money that belongs to me.
>
> I enjoy my Avon work, because I get out to meet people. I don't want to give up my freedom of meeting people. It gets me out of the house and away from the children for a little while.[2]

Secondly, paid work can meet, at least in part, women's desire for greater economic independence. Economic independence is a factor identified in studies of homeworking (Allen and Wolkowitz, 1987). It emerges, too, in studies where women leave the home to work. In a study of White married couples in the south-east of England, two-thirds of the women said that it was important to 'have some money you know is your own' (Pahl, 1989, p.130). Economic independence has been emphasised by African–Caribbean women workers. They have noted how it was the increased availability of regular waged work, denied to them in the Caribbean, that brought many of them to Britain in the 1950s and 1960s (Phizacklea, 1982; Stone 1983).

Earning your keep is an important issue for many women who live with men. It is also an issue for many lone mothers. They highlight their dual responsibilities, both to care for their children and to provide for them financially (Bradshaw and Millar, 1991). It is a responsibility that can leave them feeling deeply ambivalent about depending on the state for the money they need to live.

> I don't feel right about taking it (social security benefits). I mean I

> have to because I have no choice. . . . I just don't feel right about it, you know. Like people think, 'Oh another single parent getting everything free' and it isn't nice to be like that. But there are circumstances when you've got no choice. I mean I tried to work but it didn't pay.[3]

Economic independence is closely related to the third reason why women work. They work because they need the money. In a major survey of women's employment carried out for the Department of Employment, over a third (35 per cent) of those interviewed said that they worked primarily to earn money for essentials; another 20 per cent said they worked for money for extras (Martin and Roberts, 1984). Economic survival is also a dominant theme in homeworkers' accounts of why they work (Allen and Wolkowitz, 1987).

Financial pressures are also to the fore in studies which have focused on mothers' employment. In the Brannen and Moss study of women returning to work full time after the birth of their first baby, two-thirds gave money as the reason (Brannen and Moss, 1988). In their study, mothers' earnings represented a very substantial proportion of total household income (around 40 per cent). Where women make a relatively small contribution to the household's income, financial reasons tend to loom larger still. The survey by Martin and Roberts of women's employment found that when earnings by women represented a relatively small proportion of household income, they were most likely to see their wages as essential to the survival of their families. Those contributing 20 per cent or less to total household income were more likely to say that they could not manage financially without their earnings than those contributing 30 per cent or more (Martin and Roberts, 1984).

Women's earnings, like their unpaid labour, are typically devoted to maintaining the home and family. Surveys in the north-east of England, like those in the south-east, have noted how wives and mothers spend their wages on items related to the upkeep of the home and the care of children (Morris, 1987; Pahl, 1989). Studies of mothers returning to work after childbirth, like studies of homeworkers, have similarly found that women's earnings are devoted to essential items, including food, fuel, rent/mortgage and children's clothes (Allen and Wolkowitz, 1987; Brannen and Moss, 1988).

The conclusion that emerges from these studies is that women take on paid work in order to secure or supplement the resources they need to care for their families. For women living with men, the financial pressure to work is linked, in turn, to low pay and unemployment among men. In her study of Gujarati women in north-west London, Shrikala Warrier noted how 'with the rising levels of male unemployment and the deepening recession, the extension of women's economic functions from resource management to resource procurement has been taken almost for granted' (Warrier, 1988, p.136). A study of Punjabi Sikh women settled in West London and the Midlands suggested a similar pattern, with the unstable employment position of men resulting in a greater economic role for women (Bhachu, 1988). The importance of women's financial contribution to the household is underlined in other studies. These suggest that four times as many households would be in poverty if married women stopped going out to work (L. Morris, 1991).

However, it is not only low pay among men that has been identified as encouraging women into the labour market. Research has also pointed to women's restricted access to household income as an important factor. Being a wage earner provides women with a way of making up for shortfalls in the money they receive from their partners. Used to supplement the housekeeping money, partners can remain unaware both of their wives' need for money and of the contribution that women's wages make to keeping the family afloat (L. Morris, 1991). The ideology, if not the reality, of the family wage thus remains intact. As one respondent in Jan Pahl's study of money in marriage put it, 'he likes to think he is still running the house and is the breadwinner and my job is just an extra job I do because I want to' (Pahl, 1989, p.128).

6.4 Mothers and paid work

Women with dependent children form an increasingly significant part of the labour force. Over the last two decades, employment levels have increased more rapidly among women with dependent children than among those without (Office of Population Censuses and Surveys, 1990a). As Figure 6.1 suggests, nearly 60 per cent of women of working age with children have part- or full-time jobs. Among women without dependent children, over 70 per cent are in paid work. Among men of working age, 89 per cent have a paid job (Office of Population Censuses and Surveys, 1991a).

Not only are more mothers working but more mothers are returning to work more quickly after the birth of their baby. In the late 1980s, nearly half of the mothers who were in paid work when they became pregnant were back in employment within nine months of having their babies. A decade earlier, in the late 1970s, the proportion in paid work was only a quarter (McRae and Daniel, 1991).

While more mothers are in paid employment and are more quickly back in paid work, their employment profiles still differ markedly from women without dependent children and from men. As Figure 6.1 indicates, women with children are less likely to be in paid work or, if they do work, less likely to work full time than women without children. Women have been described as following a U-shaped employment career. They move from full-time paid work before their children are born to full-time motherhood, before re-entering the labour market as part-time workers as their children get older. It is a pattern confirmed in Figure 6.2.

Figure 6.2 suggests that only a small minority of women with preschool children (12 per cent) are in full-time work, with the

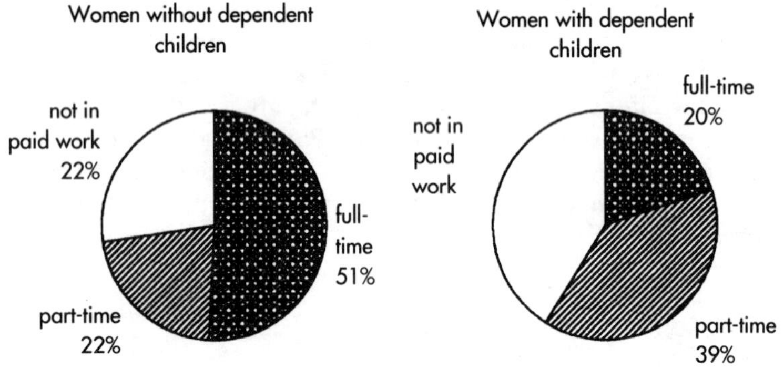

Figure 6.1 Economic activity of women aged 16 to 59 with and without dependent children, Britain, 1989.

Note: Dependent children are persons aged under 16 or aged 16 to 18 in full-time education, in the family unit and living in the household.
Source: Office of Population Censuses and Surveys (1991a), derived from Tables 3.6 and 3.7.

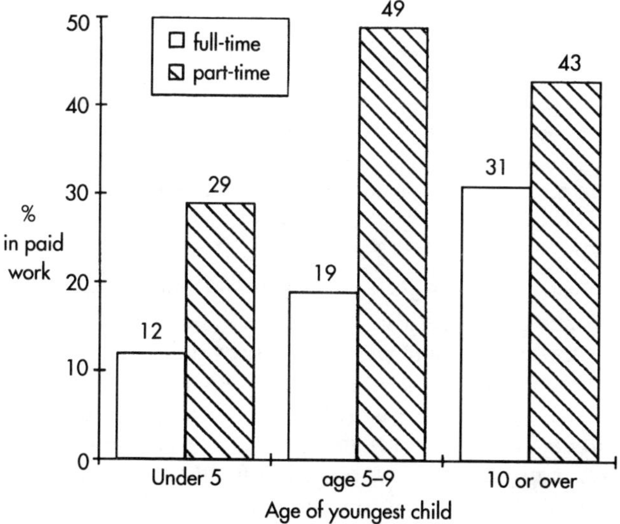

Figure 6.2 Economic activity of women of working age, proportion working full time and part time by age of youngest dependent child, Britain, 1989.

Note: Dependent children are persons under 16 or aged 16 to 18 in full-time education, in the family unit and living in the household.
Source: Office of Population Censuses and Surveys (1991a), derived from Table 3.5.

proportion increasing among women with children aged 5 to 9 (19 per cent) and among those with secondary school-aged children (31 per cent). The figure also highlights the way in which motherhood and part-time work are linked. Most working mothers with dependent children are in part-time jobs. A significant proportion of these part-time workers work in the evening or at night, at times when partners are at home. Among the women with preschool children in part-time jobs interviewed for the government's survey of women's employment, 44 per cent worked evenings or nights compared with 15 per cent of other women in part-time jobs (Martin and Roberts, 1984).

> Because the summer holidays were on the way and I had no one to look after the kids, I decided to work the 11pm to 7am shift at the

> local motorway services station. With a couple of exceptions it was all married women who worked there.
>
> Getting a good regular sleep was always a problem. We'd all go home in the morning, get the family up and off to school/work, do a bit of housework, shopping, and then prepare the evening meal. I'd go to bed till everyone got in and then get up and go to work. It was worse at weekends and when the summer holidays arrived. I'd sometimes snatch only a couple of hours sleep on a Friday morning and then not go to bed again until Sunday. During the week I dozed when the kids went out and snapped at them the rest of the time because I was so tired.[4]

While capturing overall trends, women's employment patterns are often more complex than Figures 6.1 and 6.2 suggest. Firstly, in describing employment patterns, it provides only a rough guide to mothers' employment preferences. As noted in Chapter 4, many women may prefer to look after their young children full time. Others, whether through personal preference or economic necessity, may want to stay in work after their children are born (Section 6.3). However, in the late 1980s, 40 per cent of all the employed pregnant women in Britain did not meet the employment conditions that give women a statutory right to return to work following the birth of their children (McRae and Daniel, 1991). Women in lower skilled manual jobs are particularly likely to find that they do not qualify for statutory leave. To qualify for leave, a woman who works more than 16 hours a week must have been with the same employer for at least two years. A woman working between 8 and 16 hours a week needs to have been in continuous employment with the same employer for a minimum of five years. There is no statutory provision for fathers wishing to share the care of their children.

Limited employment rights can combine with limited alternatives for childcare to keep mothers at home with their children (Moss, 1991). In a recent study of 900 working-class women with babies of six months old, the vast majority were caring for their babies full time. However, among those not in paid work, over half (57 per cent) stated that if there was someone to look after their children, they would look for part-time or full-time work (Graham, 1992a).

Secondly, Figure 6.2 suggests a standard employment pattern for mothers. However, rather than leaving the labour market once to have children and then rejoining it on a permanent basis once her children reach school age, a woman may follow a more winding career path. She may take up paid work between children, work more or less continuously while her children are young or move intermittently between paid employment and full-time care as needs and circumstances change. Repeated redundancy, particularly among Black women, is an important reason why mothers move in and out of paid work (Phizacklea, 1982).

> After my son was born . . . I gave up full-time work and went back to working part-time in the evenings. When my husband got home from work, he would look after the children while I went to work. When they were a bit older, I took up shift-work. I started at 9.00am and finished at 3.30pm, then I went back at 5.00pm and worked through until 8.00pm. I found it a great strain, but at the same time I wasn't thinking of myself. After some really bad experiences with childminders, I figured it was better to look after my own children. Then at least the children can grow up close to you and you know they are well looked after.[5]

Thirdly, Figure 6.2 does not reflect the downward drift in many women's occupational status as they move back into the labour market. While men can anticipate upgrading and promotion in the course of their working life, women need to be prepared for downward occupational mobility. Studies suggest that a significant minority of mothers re-enter the labour market through lower status jobs than the ones they held previously. Among mothers in the national survey of women's employment, for example, over a third (37 per cent) of those returning to work after the birth of their first child went into a lower level job than their previous occupation (Martin and Roberts, 1984). Another study, again based on national data, came to similar conclusions. Looking at women who had returned to work within 10 years of the birth of their first child, it found that three in ten had taken up a different kind of job which was likely to be worse paid than the one they had held before (Joshi, 1989).

> Like most women whose job is part-time, I have to put up with all sorts of bad conditions and low wages that men would never tolerate. Because I have children, work has to fit in with school hours and my husband's job. . . . A typical day for me begins at 7.30 – I get up. Wake the children. Give them breakfast. Wash up. Make the beds. 8.45 I take them to school. Come home 9.05. Clean the house. Do the washing. Go shopping. See to any bills

etc. 11.00 go to work. Come home 3.30. Collect the children from school. Make tea. Do the ironing. Prepare dinner. Eat dinner. Wash up. Go to work again at 7.00pm. Come home from work between 11.30pm and 1am, depending on how busy we are. Tidy away all the mess left by my family. Wash the dishes left lying around from the evening snacks. Make sandwiches for their packed lunches tomorrow. Go to bed.[6]

The evidence suggests that mothers often find themselves at the sharp end of economic restructuring. They are being drawn back into the labour market into more flexible and less skilled work in the service sector, for example, as part-time shop assistants and night-time cleaners. As one study concluded, 'a natural break in women's work activity over childbirth is coinciding with or being used to shift the women's workforce out of non-manual and skilled work into part-time semi-skilled work' (Dex, 1984, p.48). Flexible work, it seems, is work for women with children.

The downward drift in occupational status is a trend which impacts more on some groups of mothers than others. For example, women in professional jobs, such as nurses and teachers, are less likely to move into shop work or into semi-skilled and unskilled work after they complete their families than clerical workers. Nearly half of women in clerical jobs, but only a quarter of nurses and other professional women, moved into these occupations after they had had children (Dex, 1984). The greater protection afforded to women with professional training and experience was underlined in the study by Brannen and Moss of mothers returning to work. It was those in professional jobs and with higher qualifications who were most likely to return to work full time after the birth of their first baby and to return to their previous job (Brannen and Moss, 1988).

It is not only her previous work experiences that influence a mother's chances of finding secure and well-paid employment. Women's experiences of health and disability are also meshed into their patterns of paid work after children are born. Disabled mothers are less likely to have paid jobs than non-disabled mothers. The OPCS surveys of disability in Britain found that less than a third of married disabled women with dependent children were in paid employment (Martin and White, 1988). Among all women with dependent children, nearly 60 per cent are in paid work (see Figure 6.1). In large part, these differences reflect the fact that disabled women are much less likely to have part-time or full-time jobs than non-disabled women (see Section 6.2). However, it is also likely to reflect the difficult choices that a mother with a disability or a long term illness may have to make between keeping on caring and keeping on working for pay.

> I got depressed when I was ill this time. My first thought was for my daughter Laura and what would happen to her if I wasn't here. I always thought she would go to my sister and family in Scotland as there was something about going to my family that felt warm and secure. I thought a lot about work too. I'm sure everyone goes through this who has serious ill-health. Should I be working full-time? Should I be cutting down? Can I afford it financially? If I only have a couple of years to live should I be spending more time with Laura? . . . My two big problems are, am I going to be healthy enough to go back to work and do a good job . . . or will I make myself even iller by going back? Also I am in about eight to ten thousand pounds debt which is just about doing me in because I am not managing as it is on what I'm earning.[7]

The conflict between caring at home and working for pay is also acutely felt by many women caring for disabled children. Their lives are often more tightly meshed into the routines that support the care and development of their child than other mothers. The financial costs of childcare also tend to be greater. The needs of their disabled child mean that more is spent on food, fuel, transport, clothes and shoes, and durable household goods such as washing machines (Baldwin, 1985). While spending more than other families, the incomes of households with a disabled child are typically lower (Smyth and Robus, 1989). A major factor in the lower incomes of families with a disabled child is the fact that their mothers do not follow the patterns mapped out in Figure 6.2. Only a minority of women with disabled children return to work. As their children get older, their employment profiles diverge more and more sharply from those of other mothers with school-aged children. Among women with children over 11, women with non-disabled children are twice as likely to work as a mother with a disabled child (Baldwin, 1985). When they do go out to work, they are more likely to work fewer hours and for less pay than mothers with non-disabled children.

> My life changed radically as a result of having my children. Within four years of becoming a parent I had changed from full-time work to not doing any paid work. When I first stopped work and moved to Sheffield and started the programme (for her disabled son) I did not miss going out to work. Organising and running the programme, the ordinary aspects of bringing up two young children and the work required to keep a house going, left me with little time or energy to miss anything from my previous life. . . . Since stopping the programme, and Kim going to school full-time, I have again found myself isolated. I miss adult company. I am beginning to think about going back to work and building up my own, separate life. . . . I think about my future in a different way from my friends who have children with no disabilities. I cannot take my independence once the children are grown up for granted, as most parents do. It seems extremely unlikely that Kim will ever be completely independent. So, the possibilities of freedom for me when the children are older become less probable because I will have Kim and whatever arrangements I make for him as an adult, he will still be my dependent.[8]

Among the factors constraining the employment choices of mothers is the need to adapt their working hours to ensure that they are at home when their disabled child is not at school. This is usually done by confining paid work to term-time and to school hours. As a result, their employment opportunities are more likely to be restricted to flexible and low-paid employment, to such jobs as school-meals attendants, barmaids, and canteen and pensioner-club attendants (Baldwin, 1985).

> Normally I would be able to think of going full-time now, because when they come home from school you can find a friend or someone to take them in and look after them. Whereas no one will look after Darren. Friends are a bit nervous and frightened of handling him. They *like* him, but they just don't like to handle him. And if he holds his breath or anything like that, they just panic.[9]

While less constrained in their options, access to childcare is a major issue for parents of non-disabled children. It is an issue for mothers rather than fathers: it is mothers whose employment turns on their making appropriate arrangements for their children. Some mothers find a solution to the problem of childcare by providing it themselves. They work from home, producing goods and services for an outside employer, for the family business or for the wider community (Phizacklea, 1988). Mothers take on homesewing, they work as secretaries or bookkeepers for their partners, and they provide a range of personal services for other women, like childcare, hairdressing and running mail-order catalogues (Leira, 1987). Other mothers are able to combine childcare with paid employment outside the home, taking jobs – as nursery nurses, for example – which enable them to care and work at the same time. These kinds of solution figure strongly in Asian women's lives (Afshar, 1989).

> My mother-in-law sat at the till and my husband did all the bulk buying and shifting and that sort of thing. I could keep an eye on the children, do the cooking and cleaning and give a hand where needed. It wasn't what I had thought married life would be like. But the children needed me more than anyone else and as the shop got bigger I needed to work there as well. It was the only way we could raise the children and earn a living. Besides, at least it was my husband who was the boss and I didn't have to take orders from a stranger.[10]

While some mothers are able to resource their own childcare, the majority rely on others. The alternative sources of care are typically informal. Relatives are the major source of childcare for working women, with partners and mothers as the relatives most often involved (Martin and Roberts, 1984; Witherspoon and Prior, 1991). It is a pattern repeated among mothers with preschool children. The General Household Survey suggests that 60 per cent of mothers working full time rely on informal networks for the care of their preschool children. Partners, relatives and, for a small minority, friends and neighbours provide most of the care that enables mothers to work (Popay and Jones, 1990).

Although partners are an important resource for married women, ex-partners play only a limited part in supporting the employment of lone mothers. Bradshaw and Millar (1991) found that, among lone mothers with preschool children who were using care, only one in twenty (5 per cent) were receiving childcare from their former partners. As Table 6.1 suggests, lone mothers turn to other people in their informal network and,

Table 6.1 Type of childcare among lone mothers with preschool children using care.

Informal	%
Mother/mother-in-law	42
Other relative	18
Friend/neighbour	15
Former partner	5
Current partner	1
Older after younger	1
Formal	**%**
Childminder	18
State/LA nursery	12
Private nursery	5
Play group	4
Other	6

Note: More than one source of care is possible.
Source: Bradshaw and Millar (1991), Table 5.7.

particularly, to their mothers and other relatives. The formal sector of childcare plays a relatively limited role in helping lone mothers who wish to return to work. Faced with the difficulties of finding reliable and affordable care, lone mothers often depend on jobs which can be fitted around school hours and term-times. Like mothers with disabled children, they find themselves searching for employment in the flexible labour force, where pay is often low and job security is limited. Their employment experiences highlight the disadvantages that many mothers face in today's labour market. It is their employment patterns and experiences which are the focus of the final section of the chapter.

6.5 Patterns of employment among lone mothers

Employment trends among lone mothers are running counter to those found among married and cohabiting mothers, and among women without children. While economic activity rates among married and cohabiting mothers have been rising, rates among lone mothers have been falling. Over the last decade, the proportion of lone mothers in full-time work has shrunk, from 22 per cent in the late 1970s to 17 per cent in the late 1980s. The proportion in part-time work has also fallen slightly leaving a larger majority (60 per cent) outside the labour market (Figure 6.3). At the same time, the proportion of married mothers in both full-time and part-time work has increased. As a result, a larger majority (nearly 60 per cent) of married/cohabiting mothers is now in the labour market than was the case in the early 1980s (Office of Population Censuses and Surveys, 1990a).

The patterns of employment among lone mothers not only diverge from those found among married mothers, they also differ from the employment profile of lone fathers. Lone fathers are much more likely to be economically active and to be

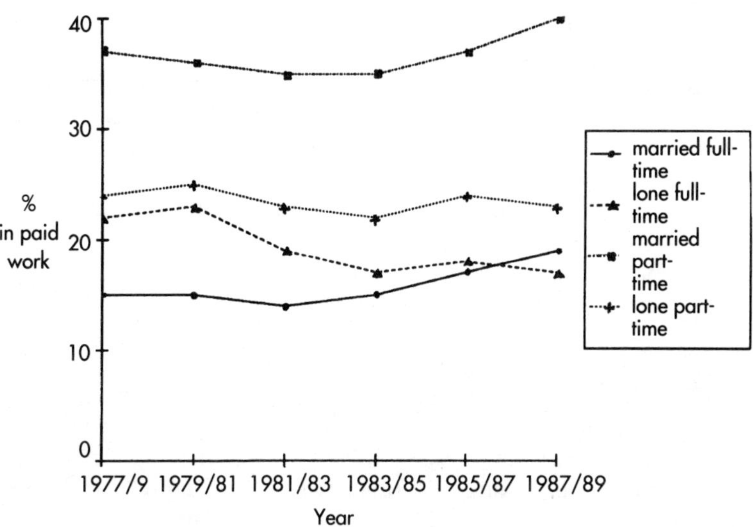

Figure 6.3 Patterns of employment among married women and lone mothers with dependent children, proportion working full time and part time, Britain, 1977–9 to 1987–9.

Note: Dependent children are persons under 16 or aged 16 to 18 and in full-time education, in the family unit and living in the household.
Source: Office of Population Censuses and Surveys (1991a), derived from Table 3.8.

employed full time. Whereas 17 per cent of lone mothers work full time and 23 per cent work part time, analyses of the Labour Force Survey indicate that 55 per cent of lone fathers are in full-time employment, with 4 per cent in part-time jobs (Haskey, 1991a). Like married women with children, this suggests that nearly 60 per cent of lone fathers are in the labour force.

Low rates of employment among lone mothers are matched by high rates of take-up of income support. Of the 1 million-plus lone mothers in Britain in the early 1990s, 774,000 relied on income support for part or all of their income (Department of Social Security, 1992a). Among the minority who are not on income support, most are in full-time work with earnings that lift them above the benefit threshold (Bradshaw and Millar, 1991).

Income support serves to highlight other lines of difference among lone mothers. Bradshaw and Millar suggest that mothers who are not dependent on benefits are typically older, ex-married women with school-age children, with more qualifications and a history of regular work. They are more likely to live in owner-occupied housing and receive maintenance. In contrast, lone mothers on income support are more likely to be younger, single women with preschool children. They have fewer qualifications and less employment experience, and are more likely to live in council accommodation and not receive maintenance (Bradshaw and Millar, 1991).

Without access to full-time work which pays enough to lift them out of poverty, lone mothers on benefit are limited in the amount they can earn before they lose a £1.00 of benefit for every £1.00 they earn. The regulations governing earnings means that they are restricted to part-time work, in which low rates of pay predominate. Further, recent changes in the treatment of childcare expenses can leave mothers on income support worse off as a result of taking part-time work (see Chapter 7). Those who find paid work are disproportionately represented in the retail, catering and cleaning sectors of the economy. In contrast to married/cohabiting women with children and to other lone mothers, the study by Bradshaw and Millar suggests that the majority (62 per cent) of employed lone mothers on benefit have jobs which involve selling, catering and cleaning. Conversely, while around a third of all women in employment are in clerical and secretarial occupations, only one in ten of the employed lone mothers on benefit in their study worked as a clerk or a secretary

(Bradshaw and Millar, 1991). Their patterns of employment are summarised in Table 6.2.

> I used to pack my job in every summer so I could fit in with the school holidays. I only did them to get some extra money so I wasn't very fussy about what I did. I never earned very much.
>
> I have to shoulder all the responsibility which means that I work because it's the only way we can survive financially. I do office cleaning late at night while my mother comes round to baby-sit. I'm lucky because I don't have to pay her anything to come round and I can catch up on my sleep when the children are at school and be at home when they come out.[11]

Table 6.2 Lone mothers in employment: mothers on and not on income support compared.

Type of job (Selected types)	On IS (%)	Not on IS (%)
Catering, retail	36	12
Domestic cleaning	26	4
Clerical, secretarial	10	38
Other service work	9	4
Nurse, teacher, skilled non-manual	5	19
Professional, manager	0	5

Source: Bradshaw and Millar (1991), Table 5.2. (Reproduced by permission of the authors)

Lone mothers experience, in a particularly acute way, the problems and pressures which confront many women with children. Financial necessity is driving more mothers to search for jobs at a time when economic restructuring is tying women's employment more firmly into the low paid and marginal sectors of the labour market. The financial circumstances of families are explored in more depth in the next chapter, which is concerned with the sources of income on which families depend for their survival.

Notes

1. Mother quoted in Pollert (1981), pp.119–20.
2. Married mother and lone mother, Graham, unpublished data.
3. Lone mother quoted in Popay (1989), p.43.

4. Taking Liberties Collective (1989), p.12.
5. Mother quoted in Bryan *et al.* (1985), p.31.
6. Taking Liberties Collective (1989), p.13.
7. Sheila in O'Sullivan and Thompson (1992), pp.28–9 and 33.
8. Murray (1992), pp.149–50 and 151–2.
9. Mother of a severely disabled boy of eight quoted in Baldwin (1985), p.79.
10. Mother quoted in Afshar (1989), p.223.
11. Two lone mothers quoted in Hardey and Glover (1991), pp.102 and 107.

CHAPTER 7

FINDING THE MONEY

7.1 Introduction

This chapter is concerned with how families find the money they need to keep themselves going. The first section explores the question of where the money comes from. It notes how it is earnings that resource most two-parent families while most lone mothers depend on state benefits. It describes the relatively minor role played by maintenance in the economic survival of lone mothers. The central two sections of the chapter look in more detail at welfare benefits and maintenance, and the changing regulations governing these sources of income. The final two sections widen the discussion of income to include credit and debt. Both occupy an increasingly important place in the domestic economy of low-income families representing, respectively, both a solution and a problem for mothers struggling to make ends meet.

7.2 Sources of income among one-parent and two-parent households

Most households with dependent children have earnings as their main source of income. In the late 1980s, two-thirds (66 per cent) of total family income came from earnings. Social security benefits made up only 14 per cent of the total income coming into families with children (Family Policy Studies Centre, 1990). As is so often the case with family statistics, these national patterns are built up out of divergent experiences. Broadly describing the income position of two-parent families, they mask the very different economic realities for one-parent families. Their different economic circumstances are summarised in Figure 7.1.

Among households with two parents, the labour market is the major source of income. As Figure 7.1 suggests, 86 per cent of their income comes from earnings. The reliance on earnings reflect the fact that most fathers with dependent children (92 per cent) are in paid work (Office of Population Censuses and Surveys, 1991a). It reflects, too, the contribution that mothers make to the income of two-parent families. Six in ten (60 per cent) of couples with dependent children are in paid work, with dual-earner households concentrated among those with older children. Although most married and cohabiting mothers work part time, their earnings make an important contribution to household income. Among dual-earner couples with children, women's earnings contribute about 25 per cent of the household's total income from employment (Family Policy Studies Centre, 1990). It is estimated that these households have weekly incomes which are 45 per cent higher than married and cohabiting

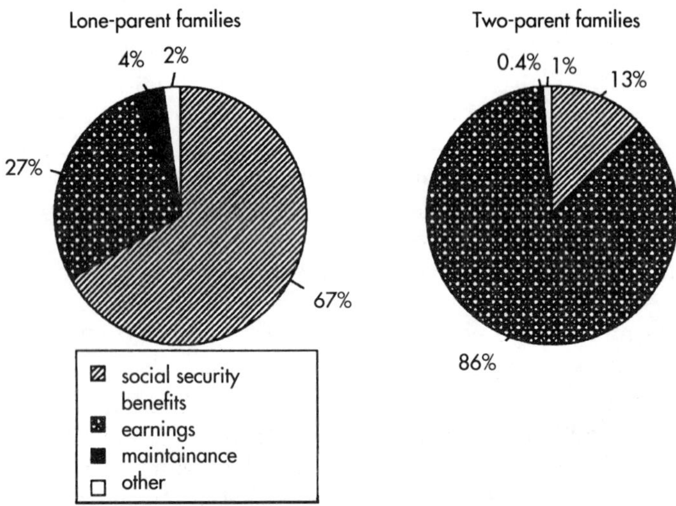

Figure 7.1 Main source of income for one-parent and two-parent households, Britain, 1987.

Source: Family Policy Studies Centre (1990), Table 1 based on House of Commons written answer 22/2/90 col. 59–60. (Courtesy of Family Policy Studies Centre)

couples with children where the mother is not in paid employment.

Among one-parent households, it is the state, not the labour market, that is the major income provider. Two-thirds (67 per cent) of the income coming into one-parent families is in the form of social security benefits. The reliance on benefits reflects the employment difficulties facing lone mothers, where limited employment opportunities and limited childcare facilities combine to make it hard for all but a small minority to earn enough to support their families (see Chapter 6).

The patterns described in Figure 7.1 capture those found in one- and two-parent families where parents and children are non-disabled. In families with disabled children, the state is a more important income source. For example, among two-parent households with a disabled child, state benefits represent 20 per cent rather than 13 per cent of average weekly income (Smyth and Robus, 1989). In families with a disabled parent, too, social security benefits make up a larger proportion of weekly household income than in other households (Martin and White, 1988).

7.3 Social security benefits

The benefit system does not function as a unified whole, operating within a single set of rules. Instead it is a set of interlocking systems, each with different regulations and practices (Roll, 1991). It includes universal (non-means-tested) benefits such as child benefit, which is the major source of independent income available to mothers. In 1991, a two-tier structure was introduced, with a higher level of benefit for the oldest eligible child. The weekly benefit in 1992/3 provided £9.65 for an only or oldest child and £7.80 for second and subsequent children.

Like other benefits, there are conditions attached to eligibility for child benefit. It is payable to the parent (or other adult) who is responsible for the child, who normally lives with him/her and who has been resident in the United Kingdom for six months. It is payable for each child up to the age of 16 and for those aged 16 to 18 in full-time education up to A levels. Child benefit is not usually paid for children who, while financially supported by a parent here, are living outside Britain. It is a condition which works against families separated by immigration control, where parents living in the United Kingdom are waiting to be reunited with their children. As Paul Gordon and Anne Newnham note, child benefit is 'reserved for those families fortunate enough to live together' (Gordon and Newnham, 1985, p.39). Within the eligibility criteria, child benefit is estimated to have a near-100 per cent take-up (Brown, 1988). The survey *Black and White Britain* found that almost all eligible Asian, African–Caribbean and White households were receiving child benefit (Brown, 1984).

Beyond this universal benefit lie the discretionary sources of state support. The most important of these is income support. which is paid to those without a full-time job who meet the conditions governing entitlement. Claimants must usually be available for and actively seeking paid employment. The exceptions include lone parents with a child under 16 and a claimant who is looking after a severely disabled person.

Access to income support and to other means-tested benefits is affected by a person's immigration status. Entitlement to income support is restricted to those who are not subject to immigration control and either have right of entry to Britain or are granted indefinite leave to stay. These eligibility criteria impact most on Black families whose entry to Britain has been determined by the increasingly restrictive regulations governing New Commonwealth immigration (see Chapter 2). People who have limited leave to stay and those whose terms of entry are subject to their having no recourse to public funds are not entitled to ordinary income support (Child Poverty Action Group, 1992). Parents, too, cannot claim for children who enter with a parent who is given limited leave: during that time, they are also subject to the public funds test and the settled parent cannot claim for them. In contrast, EC citizens can claim full income support as long as they are exercising their right to be here under the Treaty of Rome, which allows for the free movement of people within the European Community to take up employment. The effect of these different eligibility criteria is to reproduce – and reinforce – within the social security system the wider inequalities in the position of Black and White families in Britain (Gordon and Newnham, 1985; Gordon, 1991).

The social security system operates, too, in ways which reflect assumptions about the position of women and their domestic relationships with men. Assessment for benefit is based on the assumption that women either live alone or with a male partner. Lesbian and gay partners who live together do not count as a couple and are treated for benefit purposes as single people. It is one of those rare instances where unequal treatment is to the advantage of those discriminated against. It means that a woman who lives with a woman receives more income support than a woman who lives with a man. This is because once a woman and a man are judged to be a couple, they are treated as a unit, with means-testing applied to their joint resources, both capital and income, to determine the level of benefit. This assessment procedure is commonly known as the 'cohabitation rule'. The assumption underlying it is that couples pool their resources and, further, that this pooling achieves economies. Thus, the income support rate for heterosexual couples is about 60 per cent (rather than 100 per cent) higher than the rate for a single person; a heterosexual couple treated as a single unit for housing benefit purposes receives 1.6 times the benefit of a single person (Roll, 1991).

The income of families on income support is made up of two elements, as Table 7.1 suggests. Firstly, there are the personal allowances, with different rates set for cohabitating couples and lone parents and for children of different ages. For example, in 1992/3, a lone mother aged 18 with two children under 11 would receive a personal allowance for herself of £42.45 plus £14.55 for each of her children (a total of £71.55). Secondly, and in addition to the personal allowances, there are premiums. All parents receive the family premium; a lone parent also receives a lone parent premium. Thus, on top of her £71.55 personal allowances, a lone mother receives a further £14.05 a week in family and lone parent premiums, bringing her total income support to £85.60. Parents with a disabled child may be eligible for the disabled child premium and those who are registered disabled may be eligible to disability premiums. In addition, households on income support are entitled to child benefit, but this is counted as income and deducted from their income support. Income support claimants are not expected to pay their rent, which is covered by housing benefit. However, they are expected to pay 100 per cent of their water rates from their income support.

Being a woman significantly increases the chances of bringing

Table 7.1 Income support scale rates, April 1992/3. (£ sterling)

Personal allowances	£
Lone parent	
under 18 (usual rate)	25.55
under 18 (in certain circumstances)	33.60
18 or over	42.45
Couple	
both under 18	50.60
one or both over 18	66.60
Dependent children	
under age 11	14.55
age 11–15	21.40
age 16–17	25.55
age 18	33.60
Premiums	
Family premium	9.30
Lone parent premium	4.75
Disabled child premium	17.80
Disability premium	
single	17.80
couple	25.55
Severe disability premium	
single	32.55
couple (one qualifies)	32.55
couple (both qualifies)	65.10

Source: Child Poverty Action Group (1992), p.vii.

up children on the minimum levels of income provided through the benefit system. Of the 1.1 million families on income support only a third (33 per cent) contain a man. Two-thirds (66 per cent) are headed by lone mothers. This group, of 774,000, represents the majority of lone mothers in Britain (Department of Social Security, 1992a).

Figure 7.2 maps out the patterns of income support which emerged in a recent survey of 1400 lone parents (Bradshaw and Millar, 1991). It indicates that 71 per cent of lone mothers are currently dependent on income support. A higher proportion (84 per cent) have brought up their children on this minimum level of income at some time, either now or in the past. Only one in six

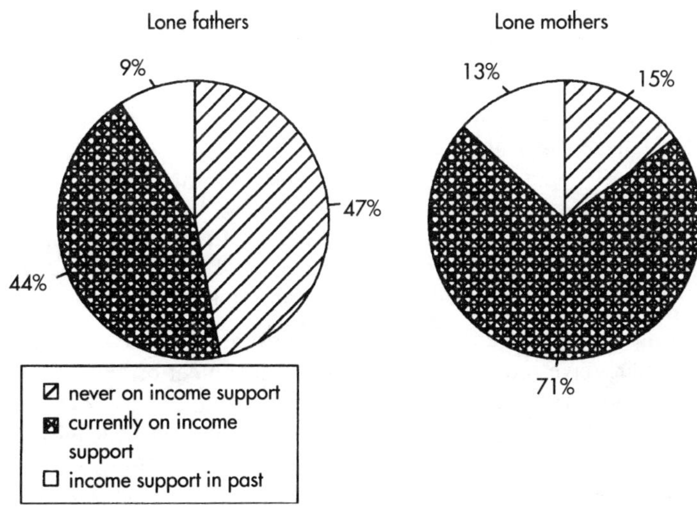

Figure 7.2 Experience of income support: lone fathers and lone mothers compared.
Source: Bradshaw and Millar (1991), derived from Table 6.2.

(15 per cent) has never been dependent on income support. In contrast, nearly half (47 per cent) of lone fathers have never relied on income support and less than one in ten (9 per cent) is currently receiving it.

Ex-married women make up the largest group of lone mothers on benefit. Over half (53 per cent) are separated and divorced mothers (Department of Social Security, 1992a). Ex-married women typically move onto benefit as a result of becoming lone mothers. In one study of separation and divorce, 15 per cent of the women were dependent on welfare benefits at the time they separated. By the time their divorce came through this proportion had risen to 46 per cent; when they were reinterviewed up to ten years later, the proportion was 56 per cent (Eekelaar and Maclean, 1985). For many lone mothers, the change in economic status, from being part of a wage-earning household to becoming a claimant, occurs at a time when their emotional resources are already taxed with the stresses and readjustments involved in splitting up.

> (I am) much, much worse off. Holidays are out, outings are out, clothes are out, drinks are out. It's just a completely different lifestyle. I just really live from month to month and just hope there's going to be enough left to cover the bills.[1]

> The worst time was when Jamie had just left and Carl would have been about two and a half, and I don't know how I coped. It was the drop in money. I'd never been to social security and it was so embarrassing. . . . I think I could have done with some sort of tranquilliser. The kids had a rotten time of it because everything went wrong and I was crying all over the house. That was dreadful but now I reckon I could cope with anything, I really do.[2]

Studies suggest that families with children, and lone mothers in particular, have more difficulty making ends meet on benefit than other types of household. Pensioner households, for example, typically report fewer problems (Berthoud, 1989). It was partly in recognition of the difficulties experienced by families with children that changes were introduced in the social security system 'to provide better targeted help for those on low incomes' (Department of Health and Social Security, 1985, p.48). The targeting metaphor, a powerful one in social security policy in recent years, suggests a system that is effective at both finding and supporting families in greatest need. However, evidence suggests that the reforms have worked to weaken rather than strengthen the financial position of families who are eligible for and rely on state benefits. This is the result of a number of interrelated trends in social security provision, three of which are highlighted here.

Firstly, there have been changes in the principles governing the uprating of benefit. Neither child benefit, nor maternity payment, a benefit designed to help women on income support to meet some of the costs of a new baby, have been uprated on an annual basis in recent years and, as a result, the monetary value of these benefits has been falling in real terms (*Maternity Action*, 1992a). The maternity payment in 1992 stood at £100. However, the government has recently committed itself to making child benefit inflation-proof, increasing it in line with rises in the cost of living (Ditch *et al.*, 1992).

The principles governing the uprating of income support were also changed in the 1980s. Rates are no longer linked to earnings but are uprated in line with prices. The effect has been to widen the gap between average incomes and the incomes of claimants. By the late 1980s, the income support received by a two-parent family with two children under 11 represented only 30 per cent of the disposable income of the average two-parent, two-child family (Bradshaw, 1990).

Secondly, combined with changes introduced earlier in the decade, the 1986 Social Security Act increased the financial responsibilities of parents on benefit. The 1986 Act removed the right to income support for most 16- and 17-year-olds, on the assumption that their parents should and could meet the costs of their care. It has hit households on benefit hard and has been identified as a major factor in the increase of rooflessness among young people (Thornton, 1990). It has also hit young pregnant women. Pregnant 16- and 17-year-olds are not normally entitled to benefit until the twenty-ninth week of their pregnancy and then receive a lower rate of benefit than those over 18 (*Maternity Action*, 1992b). The 1986 Act increased the financial responsibilities of claimants in other ways. It made it a requirement that claimants pay 100 per cent of their water rates and 20 per cent of their rates/poll tax. Under the new council tax, introduced in 1993 to replace the poll tax, the minimum contribution of 20 per cent has been abolished.

Thirdly, changes in the social security system have had the effect of reducing parents' access to additional sources of financial support from the state. For example, when income support replaced supplementary benefit in April 1988, work expenses, including childcare, could no longer be offset against part-time earnings before these counted against benefit entitlement. The evidence suggests that this change has hit lone mothers particularly hard. As a result of their childcare costs, they can be worse off as a result of taking part-time work (Bennett, 1992).

The changes in the system of single payments provides another, and more significant, example of the withdrawal of financial help from the state. Through the 1980s, single payments were the most important additional source of money for claimants. They were lump-sum grants for items that claimants were unable to meet from their regular benefit. It was families with children who turned most to single payments, reflecting the fact that they faced more additional needs and special expenses that they could not meet from their weekly benefit than other households. Single payments provided a particularly important safety-net for lone mothers (Cohen, 1988).

Through the 1980s, there was a gradual tightening of the rules governing single payments and under the 1986 Social Security Act the system was abolished. It was replaced in 1988 by a new scheme, the social fund. Because the social fund offers much more limited help through grants, most parents on benefit have to look to discretionary, interest-free loans to cope with large items of expenditure or with an emergency. The social fund offers two kinds of loans, crisis loans and budgeting loans. Crisis loans can be applied for by those who have insufficient resources to meet their 'immediate short-term needs' as the regulations governing the social fund put it. Applications for budgeting loans are restricted to claimants who have been on income support for at least 26 weeks. Loans are repaid by deductions from benefit.

> In the past, when I had my first daughter, if you were in desperate need of something they'd give you X amount and that was it. But what they do now, they ask you to take this loan and it's not so much them actually giving you the money, it's you owe money now that you haven't got.[3]

Evidence from the first few years of the social fund suggests that it is not meeting its aim of helping 'with claimants' budgeting difficulties and financial crises' (Department of Health and Social Security, 1985, p.118). Claimants, particularly Asian claimants, may know little about how the scheme works and may be reluctant to become indebted to outside agencies (G. Craig, 1991; Sadiq-Sangster, 1991; Cohen *et al*, 1992). Those seeking a loan have been refused because, ironically, their incomes are too low to cover the costs of repayments. For claimants granted a social fund loan, it can prove to be a form of debt that is too expensive. While interest-free, repayments can be pitched above what parents can afford, leaving them looking to other sources of credit to cover the shortfall (Craig and Glendinning, 1990; Cohen, 1991b).

> Before they would give you money for things you desperately needed. Now you have to get a loan and I can't afford to pay it back. . . . I don't agree with the loans, the problem is paying them back and I don't get enough.[4]

> At first I thought I might get it (budgeting loan) for the settee but then I thought if they cut any more off the £70 I already get and I can't really manage now, how will I manage with less? So I thought no, if they cut it then I would have to borrow more.[5]

Rather than increasing parents' economic independence, studies tracking the impact of the new social security regulations point to increasing debt (Cohen *et al.*, 1992). They point, too, to multiple debt problems, with money owed to a variety of different creditors and claimants forced to borrow more in order to service the repayments on debts they have already accumulated. Along with more debts has gone a 'transfer of dependency' as mothers turn from the benefit system to other sources of income, like money-lenders and relatives, for the money they need to survive (Craig and Glendinning, 1990).

> There's nothing left by the time I pay my way. I'm only on £84 a week so you can imagine how much I've got to spend on food for the rest of the week, plus my electricity, my gas, this, that and the other. Sometimes I only have a tenner left out of my giro. Sometimes I don't even have that. We don't like (to borrow) but we've got to do it, haven't we? Yes, it's the only way people get by – continuously borrowing.[6]

Credit is deeply woven into the financial strategies – and the financial problems – of mothers on low incomes. In contrast, maintenance provides relatively little of the money which mothers need to survive. However, as the next section indicates, it has become a major focus of social security policy in Britain.

7.4 Maintenance

It is the mother who usually takes responsibility for the care of children after separation and divorce (see Chapter 2). The role of fathers is typically a more limited one. Through the 1980s, the trend in Britain, and elsewhere in Europe, was towards limiting the financial liability of men to maintain their ex-families (Millar, 1989). In England and Wales, settlements were framed on the assumption that the man had only limited financial responsibilities towards his ex-wife. Maintenance, as a result, was largely defined in terms of an ex-husband's financial contribution towards the support of his children. Reflecting this emphasis on children rather than ex-partners, the Department of Social Security (DSS) expected absent parents to pay maintenance for their children up to the level of the child scale rates for income support, plus the family and lone parent premiums (see Table 7.1) (Bradshaw and Millar, 1991).

The evidence suggests that maintenance payments rarely meet the expectations laid down in law and in DSS procedures. Studies record that a significant minority of divorced mothers (around one-third) do not receive maintenance awards (Eekelaar and Maclean, 1985). Where awards are made, they are often low and well below the scale rates for children in households on income support (Millar, 1989). These findings have been confirmed by Bradshaw and Millar in their study of lone parents. Four in ten (40 per cent) of the divorced mothers received regular maintenance payments; among single mothers, the proportion was 14 per cent. The average payment per child was £16 a week, well below the expected levels of maintenance set by the DSS (Bradshaw and Millar, 1991). Reflecting these levels of payment, maintenance contributed only 7 per cent of the net income of the lone parents in the study.

The study sheds light on why levels of maintenance are generally low (Table 7.2). Of the lone mothers not receiving maintenance, one in five (20 per cent) said they did not want to

Table 7.2 Lone mothers' reasons for not receiving maintenance payments.

	%
Prefer not to receive money	20
Ex-partner is unemployed	15
He cannot afford to pay	14
Do not know where he is	14
He refused to make payments	11
Other reason	9
Don't need any	1
Don't know reason	24

Note: More than one answer is possible.
Source: Bradshaw and Millar (1991), Table 7.2.

receive payments from their ex-partners. Such a response should be set in the context of the survey's findings about the factors which contributed to the breakdown of relationships. As noted in Chapter 2, violence was cited as a reason for not living together by 20 per cent of the respondents; 16 per cent noted alcohol and drug addiction as major or contributory factors.

Table 7.2 suggests that around three in ten (29 per cent) of the lone parents who were not receiving maintenance did not regard their ex-partners as being in a position to make a financial contribution, because they were unemployed and/or because they could not afford to. Underlying these judgements are patterns in divorce which make it a more common experience for men on the margins of the labour market. Divorce rates are higher among men in semi-skilled and unskilled occupations and, particularly, among unemployed men and younger men in these occupational groups. The partners of women who have children outside marriage, too, tend to be very disadvantaged within the labour market, clustered in occupations where pay is low and the risk of redundancy is high (Chapter 2).

> I'm entitled to it [maintenance] but I don't get it because my ex-husband never sends it and now he's on the social security himself. He's gone through his second divorce and is looking after two little girls.

> I don't want it [maintenance]. It was a condition that if he disappeared out of my life and I wouldn't give him access, he wouldn't have to pay me any money. It was so rough towards the end that I was so glad just to be able to get things together.[7]

The findings summarised in Table 7.2 suggest that the scope for increasing the role that maintenance plays in the financial support of lone mothers may be limited. However, recent legislation has sought to break with norms governing maintenance in the 1980s and extend the financial liability of the absent parent. Extending the liability of fathers, in turn, represents a way of increasing the financial dependence of mothers on their ex-partners rather than on the state (Lister, 1991). The 1990 Social Security Act extended the liability of ex-spouses to include the maintenance of parents on income support who were caring for children. This financial liability was also defined to include unmarried parents. The Act imposed a duty on fathers to support the mother of his children as long as she is claiming income support and whether or not he is, or ever was, married to her.

The extension of maintenance to include both ex-spouses and ex-partners has been ratified in the Child Support Act 1991. This gives greater power to the DSS (Department of Social Security), in the person of the Secretary of State, to initiate an application for maintenance, even if the claimant wishes to have no further contact with the absent parent. It has established a Child Support Agency to deal with claims for maintenance, to trace absent parents and enforce payments of maintenance. Through the offices of the agency, it is a requirement that the caring parent makes a claim for maintenance. The DSS has the potential power to withhold benefit from women who do not wish to name the father of their child. However, the Act lays down a set of circumstances in which it is legitimate for the mother to refuse to comply with this requirement. Section 6(2) of the Child Support Act stipulates that action will not be taken to recover child support maintenance from the absent parent where there are 'reasonable grounds for believing that . . . there would be a risk to her, or of any child living with her, suffering harm or undue distress as a result'. As critics have noted, much depends on how sensitively Child Benefit Support Officers interpret this safeguard and exercise their considerable discretion (Land, 1992).

Most lone mothers and their children will gain nothing financially from the pursuit of maintenance. For the 70 per cent of lone mothers on income support, maintenance payments will continue, as at present, to be deducted from benefit. Women floated off income support because their newly received maintenance payments lifts them above the benefit threshold may well be worse off, because of the loss of passport benefits (such as the waiving of prescription charges and some other health charges, access to free school meals and social fund community care grants) for which maintenance payments might not compensate (Morton, 1991).

The new legislation is unlikely to help lone mothers tackle their financial problems. Instead, they may find themselves increasingly immersed in a complex web of credit commitments and debt repayments as they struggle to care for their children.

7.5 Consumer credit

Earnings, benefits and maintenance represent sources of current income. However, people have increasingly looked beyond these sources for the money they need to live. They have looked, particularly, to loans. Credit is the term commonly used to describe the money people borrow. It provides a way of meeting current needs out of future income, with goods, services and money received in advance of payment. About 80 per cent of outstanding credit is associated with borrowing for housing, with building societies the largest source of mortgages (Ford, 1991). Consumer credit, which covers other types of credit, like mail order catalogues and credit cards, is on a much smaller scale. However, like borrowing through mortgages, consumer credit has grown significantly over the last decade. Surveys suggest that just under half (48 per cent) of adults had credit commitments in 1979. By 1989, this had risen to 60 per cent (Berthoud and Kempson, 1992). It is estimated that a third of all consumer goods are brought on credit and that the servicing of consumer credit consumes 7 per cent of average household income (Berthoud, 1989; Berthoud and Kempson, 1992). The signs are that the 1980s boom in consumer credit is over, with figures for 1990 and 1991 showing a plateauing out in the rise of credit commitments (Berthoud and Kempson, 1992).

There are four broad categories of consumer credit. The largest sector is commercial credit, covering credit cards and overdraft facilities, mail order catalogues and hire purchase arrangements with retailers. State credit, in the form of budgeting loans from the social fund, is a relatively small credit sector and, as noted in Section 7.3, directed at households on income support. Alongside the legally regulated sources of credit, is the unregulated market of loan-sharks and money-lenders. Beyond these three sectors of credit is informal credit, where money is lent by relatives and friends.

A recent UK study sheds light on the patterning of credit commitments among households (Berthoud and Kempson, 1992). It suggests that age is an important influence, with younger adults being significantly more likely to enter into credit agreements than older adults and those over retirement age. Household income is also structured into the take-up of credit, but in a more complex way. The study suggests that a similar proportion of households across the income range use credit, ranging from 67 per cent among households on the lowest incomes to 76 per cent among the highest income households. However, they use different kinds of credit and they use credit for different reasons.

(*i*) *Different kinds of credit*

Income is linked to access to credit, with higher income households using forms of 'up-market' credit, offering a wide choice of facilities and competitive rates of interest. It is better-off households which are more likely to have a bank account and an overdraft facility, and to have credit cards and store cards. In the higher income ranges, 40 per cent of households have credit cards (Berthoud and Kempson, 1992). Low-income households typically have more restricted access to credit and rely on more expensive forms of credit. Some may be excluded altogether (Ford, 1991).

> It was somewhere down town, exactly the same washing machine and it was £100 cheaper and I thought, oh, I could have that (on hire-purchase). Well I went down, went to a few shops. . . . The first thing they ask you is, like, are you single? yes; children? yes; Social? yes: oh you can't have it.[8]

Mail-order catalogues are the most common form of consumer credit among low-income households. Catalogues are used by 45 per cent of households on the lowest incomes. In comparison, only 10 per cent have credit cards (Berthoud and Kempson, 1992). Mail-order catalogues are a particularly important source of credit for White women with children. The evidence suggests that, reflecting a more general reticence about commercial credit among Asian families, Asian mothers are less likely to use mail-order catalogues (Sadiq-Sangster, 1991).

Mail-order catalogues provide a way of purchasing items mothers need for their children, such as clothes, shoes, toys and presents, with both catalogues and goods delivered to the home (Bradshaw and Holmes, 1989; Craig and Glendinning, 1990). Catalogues are often run through family and friendship networks, with repayments structured around the weekly budgeting arrangements which operate in low-income households. Catalogues can offer a more flexible system of credit than commercial and state loans: because mothers know the agent, it can be possible to postpone and renegotiate weekly payments (Cohen, 1991a;b).

> Some of the things are expensive (in the catalogue), a lot more than you'd pay in the shops, but if it's easier for you to pay £20 extra but pay it weekly, it works out better . . . if I do ever miss a week, which I try not to do, she (neighbour who is the agent) will put it in for me and then I give it back.[9]

There are other sources of credit which specialise in meeting the credit needs of poor parents. These include the major source of state credit, the social fund (discussed in the last section), check-traders, 'tick' credit and money-lenders.

Check trading is credit given by shops up to a fixed amount, with each purchase deducted from the check and repaid by fixed weekly instalments, often across a six-month period. An important source of credit in the early 1980s, recent surveys point to a shift away from check trading towards other forms of credit among low income families (Ford, 1991).

'Tick' credit is a more informal credit arrangement that is typically made with a local shop where the mother is a known and regular customer. It remains an important source of financial help for families struggling to make ends meet, particularly for food and clothes. Most of the Asian claimants in Cohen and Sadiq-Sangster's study of families on benefit were able to buy goods on credit from local Asian shops where they were known and where they had shown loyalty to the shopkeeper (Cohen, 1991a; Sadiq-Sangster, 1991). As the parents in their study noted, the process of buying on tick is typically an ongoing one, with a cycle of debt in which last week's purchases are paid off before buying this week's food.

Like 'tick', unlicensed money-lending is a form of credit predominantly used by those on low incomes. While little is known about this credit sector, the evidence suggests that interest rates are high and can be extortionate. For example, a lone parent in the UK study of credit and debt had borrowed £100 and was paying £6.50 a week for a year: an annual rate of interest of over 200 per cent (Berthoud and Kempson, 1992). The inevitable consequence of these super-charged loans is that debtors are unable to repay the interest and this is added to the loan. They thus find themselves in an ever-climbing spiral of debt. Because illegal money lenders cannot recover money owed to them through the courts, some resort to a variety of illegal practices to ensure repayment of loans, including the holding of benefit books, and the threat and use of violence (Bolchever *et al.*, 1990). A study in Strathclyde suggested that many of those using loan-sharks were lone mothers, particularly those who already had debts relating to rent arrears and fuel bills, and were thus unable to obtain credit from a reputable source.

> The fear will always be inside me on Friday nights even though my loans are cleared now. Well, I've gone through a lot in my life, my husband being an alcoholic and my daughter having spina bifida. But I can honestly say that the worst feelings I ever had were over the money lending – that was definitely the worst thing that ever happened to me.[10]

Beyond the legal and illegal sources of credit is the informal help provided by families and friends. Studies have pointed to how families, and mothers in particular, are an important source of financial help in emergencies. In one study of two-parent families on benefit, two-thirds of the respondents said that they would turn to their families for money in an emergency. Mothers were the single most frequently cited source of help (Bradshaw and Holmes, 1989).

> Our mum, she's been ever so good, we'll go and see her and she'll say, 'Oh take a couple of pounds of sugar or a quarter of tea' . . . or a couple of 50p's for the cleaners and she's helped with other clothes for the children. My mum's not well off, not by a long way but she's tried hard to help . . . but it makes you feel guilty. . . . We don't like accepting it. It's not a situation we like but there's times when we've just had to sort of swallow our pride and say 'Thanks very much'.[11]

(ii) Credit for different reasons

Low-income households have a very different pattern of credit use than better-off households. High-income households tend to use credit to buy consumer durables, such as cars, televisions and videos, while low-income households use credit to cover the costs of surviving. Credit is taken out to pay off debts, pay bills and make ends meet (Berthoud and Kempson, 1992). It is typically regarded not as a choice but as a necessity.

> Well, I think it's desperation. I'm so desperate or else who else wants to borrow or get loans. Now you can go and see my beds upstairs. I have four children and sleeping on those two single beds, cramped in with them, it just breaks your back. Honestly, I thought and thought about buying it (a bed). If I didn't need it, honestly I wouldn't have bought it, only because I was so desperate did I get it.[12]

High-income households spend most on credit; low-income households spend least. However, it is low-income households who devote the highest proportion of their disposable income to servicing credit commitments. They do so, too, on a household income where most of their money is already devoted to meeting basic household costs, such as food, fuel and housing. As a result, those on the lowest incomes have credit commitments that exceed their available income (Berthoud and Kempson, 1992). In other words, credit is simultaneously a debt, a financial commitment that families can not meet within their weekly income.

7.6 Debt

Debt represents a financial commitment that is hard to pay. Like credit, it is a broad category and covers arrears on household costs, such as rent, mortgages and fuel bills, and arrears and overdrafts on consumer credit. There are only limited statistics on the patterns of debt over time; however, they point to an upward trend over the last decade. It has been calculated that there were around 1.3 million households with current arrears in 1981 (Berthoud, 1989). By 1989, the estimated figure stood at 2.8 million, more than double the 1981 figure (Berthoud and Kempson, 1992). Most debts relate to household expenses. Debts on housing, fuel and poll tax, and other household commitments account for two-thirds of all debts in the United Kingdom. The remaining third of debts are the result of not keeping up with consumer credit commitments (Berthoud and Kempson, 1992).

Among these different kinds of debt, it is rent arrears that are the most common debt. Despite the rise in repossessions among homeowners, the evidence suggests that the risk of debt is far greater among tenants than mortgagors, at all income levels.

It is low-income households who are at greatest risk of falling into debt. However, the risks of debt are not equally borne by all low-income households. Life-cycle position shapes which low-income families are most likely to have debt problems. Being young and having children makes people more vulnerable, with younger and larger families having more debts than older and smaller families (Berthoud, 1989; Berthoud and Kempson, 1992). Lone mothers are known to be particularly vulnerable, both to debt and to multiple debt. For some lone mothers, debt is a problem which they inherited from their previous relationship, the backdrop against which their experience of becoming a lone mother and becoming a claimant is set.

> When he left me, he left me with a lot of debts. We had a joint account and my husband ran up – well a large overdraft. I gradually managed to pay that off but I couldn't afford the standing charge. So I shut it (bank account) down. I've paid off the debts but he also left me with a lot of HP. Like an idiot, when we bought the settee, I put it in my name so it's not even in his name so I am left with it. £20 a month I'm paying, and with the interest it'll take me 10 years to pay.[13]

Once low-income families get into difficulties with repayments, the evidence suggests that they find it hard to get out of debt. The majority (over 70 per cent) who start the year in debt also end it in debt (Berthoud and Kempson, 1992). Among benefit households with children, borrowing to meet family and financial commitments has become a fact of life. In one study of two-parent families on benefit, 96 per cent were in debt, with debts averaging £441. The average weekly repayments represented 12 per cent of their weekly incomes (Bradshaw and Holmes, 1989). In a more recent survey of Asian, African–Caribbean and White families on benefit, two-thirds had debts, most commonly for housing, fuel and children's clothes (Cohen, 1991a).

> It's a vicious circle . . . you can't seem to get out of. Because the poor are kept poor. . . . You end up paying more back, whereas somebody with a bit more money is able to pay cash or a big

> deposit and they haven't got so many bills. So you have to incur debt to live.[14]

Highlighting the scale of debt among claimants, recent studies have also drawn attention to the toll it takes on their mental health. Knowing you cannot make ends meet and have to borrow to survive brings with it a particular and acute kind of anxiety: for many parents, it is one overlaid by the stigma of not managing independently. Shame about one's enforced dependence, and embarrassment that relatives and friends could find out (or know already) are dominant themes in the accounts of Black and White parents in debt (Daly, 1988; Ford, 1988; Sadiq, 1991; Sadiq-Sangster, 1991).

> Sometimes when the MEB (Electricity Board) say absolutely no, when they say that if you don't pay £150 and something then we will come and disconnect you straight away, then I go and ask from someone, I will say please help me. I have to become very humble and ask to borrow some money. And sometimes someone will give it to you or not. So it is very hard to ask anybody for money. I have to become very humble.[15]

Shame and embarrassment means that the burden of debt is often hidden within the household, shouldered by parents at a significant cost for family relationships. It can be a burden that a mother bears alone, a stigma she feels she must keep from her partner. Not surprisingly, studies have recorded how relationships between partners and with children deteriorate as parents struggle to cut back (Daly, 1988; Ford, 1988). Although reluctant to ask for money from kin, the evidence suggests that many families in debt do (Ford, 1991; Sadiq-Sangster, 1991; Berthoud and Kempson, 1992).

> My husband doesn't know (about the loans). I'm always living in dread that he's going to find out, he has to some day. He knows that the man calls every Friday but I tell him that I'm paying my friend's TV money for her. My next door neighbour tries to get her husband into her house when the money-lender is around so that he won't notice anything. He knows the book is there but I told him it belongs to my friend. I feel so guilty about not being able to manage and I don't want him to know.[16]

The evidence on debt paints a grim picture of life among

families on low incomes. It suggests that incomes among households with children at the bottom of the income scale are often insufficient to meet needs. The question of how mothers try to look after their families in such circumstances is the focus of the next chapter.

Notes

1. Lone mother quoted in Graham (1985), p.112.
2. Lone mother, unpublished data from Graham (1985).
3. Lone mother on income support quoted in Cohen (1991b), p.34.
4. Lone mother on income support interviewed in Craig and Glendinning (1990), p.39.
5. Single parent on income support quoted in Cohen (1991a), p.5.
6. Parent on benefit with four children quoted in Berthoud and Kempson (1992), p.108.
7. Lone mothers, Graham, unpublished data.
8. Lone mother on income support quoted in Cohen (1991b), pp.33–4.
9. Lone mother on income support quoted in Cohen (1991b), p.33.
10. Parent quoted in Daly (1988), p.73.
11. Married mother on benefit with two children quoted in Ritchie (1990), p.50.
12. Parent quoted in Sadiq-Sangster (1991), p.2.
13. Lone mother on benefit, Graham, unpublished data.
14. Mother on income support quoted in Cohen (1991b), p.29.
15. Parent quoted in Sadiq-Sangster (1991), p.2.
16. Married mother quoted in Daly (1988), p.74.

CHAPTER 8

MAKING ENDS MEET

8.1 Introduction

The evidence reviewed in the last chapter indicated that many families are trying to survive on very little. The trends in credit and debt among low-income households suggest that, for an increasing number, very little is not enough.

This chapter looks in a more focused way at this sense of barely surviving. It begins by looking at what official statistics suggest about the financial position of households with children, noting how many are living on incomes which make it hard to survive. It then describes how low-income families spend the limited money they have. The second part of the chapter explores what it means to experience motherhood as a conflict between health and debt, where individual well-being is constantly pitted against the financial survival of the family. It identifies some of the strategies that mothers develop as they work to keep their families in health and out of too much debt.

8.2 Families on low income

Income inequalities in Britain widened significantly through the 1970s and 1980s, with the gap between the living standards of rich and poor households growing steadily wider (O'Higgins, 1989; House of Commons, 1991). There is evidence, too, that the poorest households are not only losing out relatively but are becoming poorer in absolute terms as well. Households on the lowest incomes saw their real income (after housing costs) fall by 6 per cent between 1979 and 1989 (Department of Social Security, 1992b).

Households with children have been particularly hard hit by these widening income inequalities. They are increasingly to be found among the households whose income is falling behind the rest of the population (O'Higgins, 1989; Department of Social Security, 1992b). Their vulnerability is starkly summarised in statistics on households with incomes below 50 per cent of average income, the measure often taken as the EC poverty line. Figure 8.1 records the number of children in households with incomes which have fallen below this level over the last decade. It suggests that the number of children in poor households doubled in the course of the 1980s, from 1.6 million in 1979 to 3.1 million in 1989 (House of Commons, 1991; Department of Social Security, 1992b). Today, one in four children (25 per cent) are growing up in households below the unofficial poverty line.

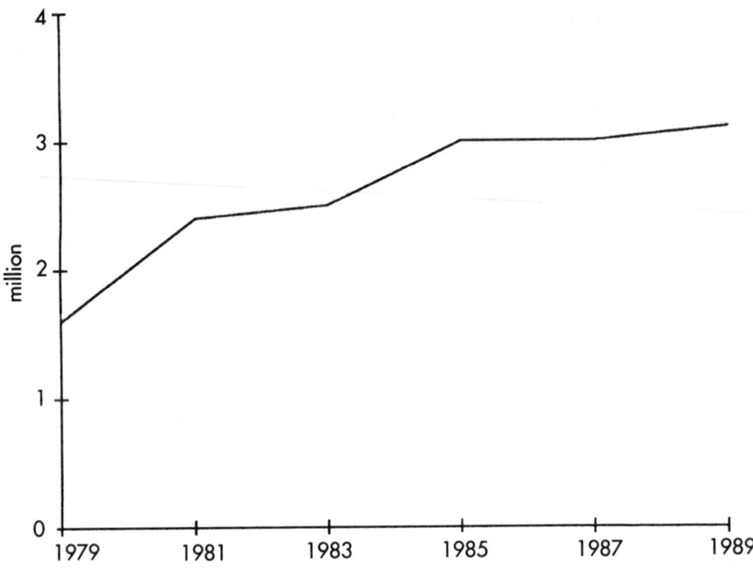

Figure 8.1 Number of dependent children in households with below 50 per cent of average income, Britain, 1979–89.

Note: Income is net of housing costs.
Source: House of Commons (1991), derived from Table F3 (1979–88 data) and Department of Social Security (1992b), derived from Table F3 (1989 data).

The burden of hardship is not one borne equally by all families, however. It is parents on the margins of the labour market whose children find their way into the statistics represented in Figure 8.1. Over a third of children in households with incomes below 50 per cent of the average have parents who 'earn their poverty': in full-time work but with earnings that put them below the poverty threshold. Another third are in households headed by parents who are unemployed and a quarter are in one-parent families. The remainder – about 8 per cent – are in households headed by a parent who is retired, sick or disabled (Oppenheim, 1990).

Counting up how many poor children come from different types of households does not, of course, tell us which children face the greatest risks of poverty. These risks are spelled out in Figure 8.2. It points to the particular vulnerability of children in

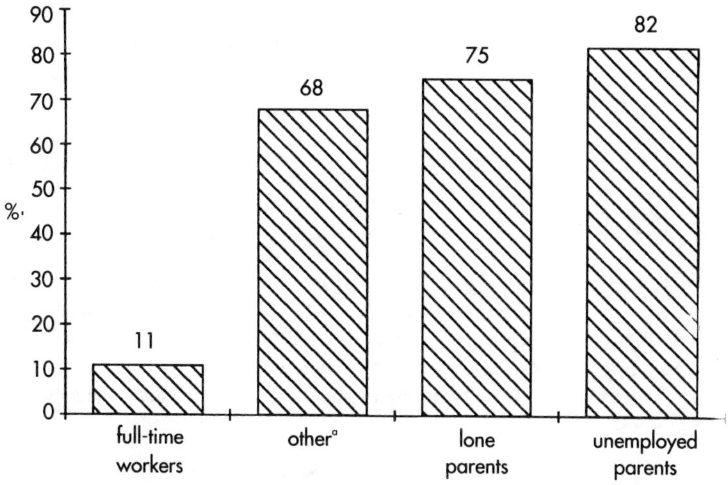

Figure 8.2 Proportion of dependent children in households with below 50 per cent of average income, by economic status of head of household, Britain, 1988.

[a] Other: pensioners, sick/disabled parents.

Notes: 1. The definition of full-time work is 24 hours or more a week. 2. Lone parents working full-time are recorded as full-time workers. 3. Income is net of housing costs.

Source: House of Commons (1991), derived from Table F3.

households headed by parents who are pensioners or disabled/ sick, by unemployed parents and by lone parents who are not in full-time work. The figure indicates that the vast majority of children in these households are being cared for on poverty-line incomes, below a level which sustains health and enables individuals to live within the communities of which they feel part.

Figure 8.2 suggests that the risks of poverty are high among households headed by a parent who is not in full-time work. For households headed by an unemployed parent, these risks have not increased very much over the last decade. However, during the 1980s, an increasing proportion of children in one-parent households and in households headed by a disabled parent or pensioner found themselves in households below the 50 per cent threshold. As a House of Commons report put it, 'children in lone parent families and in households headed by a sick/ pensioner/other adult are . . . increasingly in households whose income is falling behind that of the rest of the population' (House of Commons, 1991, p.vii). In 1979, 45 per cent of children in families headed by a lone parent were in households with below 50 per cent of the average income: in 1988, the proportion was 75 per cent. Among children in households headed by a parent who was sick, disabled or a pensioner, the proportion in households below the 50 per cent threshold rose from 40 per cent in 1979 to 68 per cent in 1988 (House of Commons, 1991).

> We're not living, we're just existing barely. . . . going into the butcher's and asking, you got some bones for my dog? And then making a pot of soup. . . . Living is where I could go into a shop and say I'll have a pound of steak, my bairns fancy a bit of steak for their tea. Or, I'd like a pair of shoes, fit them on my bairns and we'll take them.[1]

For families with incomes below the EC decency threshold, the struggle to make ends meet is typically fought out in and against the routines that sustain health. As the accounts above record, it is a struggle fought out through the routines of buying bones from the butcher and not buying shoes for the children. How families, and mothers in particular, set about the task of surviving is explored in the next three sections.

8.3 Spending in low income households

Better-off households typically budget by the month and use a bank account; low-income households budget by the week and deal in cash (Berthoud, 1989; Berthoud and Kempson, 1992). All households, however, tend to adopt a common budgeting cycle, in which financial commitments to external agencies, such as housing and fuel costs, are met before money is spent on food and other household items. Commitments to external agencies usually come in the form of fixed costs, where neither the timing nor the amount of payment can be controlled to any major extent by the household. This system of paying fixed costs first is formalised in the standing orders that better-off families set up with their banks. For low-income households, the prioritising of external commitments is more likely to be formalised through the benefit system.

Over the last decade, the external financial commitments of low-income families have increasingly become incorporated in the payment of benefits. For example, until 1983, the supplementary benefit that families received included an element for housing costs. Since the introduction of housing benefit, housing costs like rent are deducted from benefit before it is paid to the claimant. For those on income support, social fund loans and mortgage interest are paid in the same way. Many claimants, too, pay their fuel bills as direct deductions from benefit. These direct payment arrangements have the effect of reducing disposable income, leaving claimants and other households on low incomes with less flexibility about how they spend their money.

Flexibility is also restricted by the need to meet other fixed costs early in the cycle of weekly budgeting. Figure 8.3 gives an indication of the burden that these costs place on the finances of low-income households. It suggests that the richest households spend 21 per cent of their net income on household costs of various kinds, including mortgage, rent, local taxes, telephone and fuel. Another 7 per cent goes on repayments for credit and debt commitments. However, in the poorest households, the proportion of weekly income going to these external agencies is nearly twice as high. As Figure 8.3 records, households on the lowest incomes devote over half of their net weekly income to basic household costs and credit commitments.

The patterns described in Figure 8.3 suggest that only half of the money coming into poor households is available for spending on items directly related to everyday health needs, including

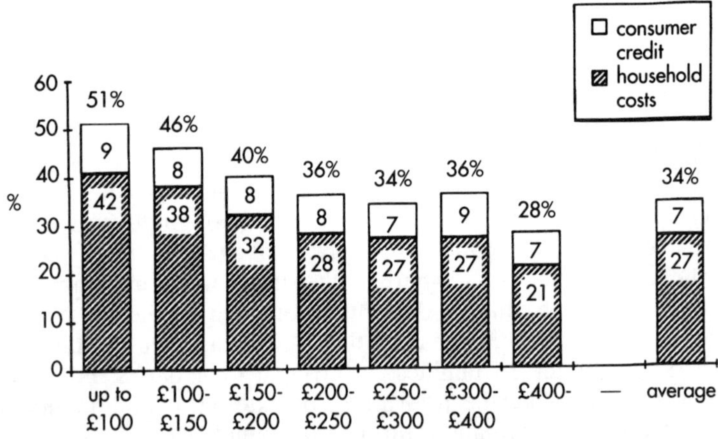

Figure 8.3 Proportion of weekly income devoted to housing costs and services, and to consumer credit, by income, United Kingdom, 1989.

Note: Household costs include mortgage, rent and associated charges, local taxes, electricity, gas and telephone.
Source: Berthoud and Kempson (1992), derived from Tables 7.1 and 7.2.

food, clothes and shoes. Independent of any controlling influence that their partners may exercise over their access to money, mothers thus find themselves working to care for their families on a significantly reduced income. It is within this income that cutbacks have to be made if spending is to be contained.

Food occupies a particularly central place in the budgeting strategies of low-income families. Firstly, it is the largest single item of household spending and low-income households spend proportionately more of the little they have on this essential health resource. The patterns of spending recorded in Table 8.1 suggest that two-parent families on benefit spend 30 per cent of their weekly income on food (Bradshaw and Holmes, 1989). Other studies have suggested that the proportion devoted to food by claimant families is higher still, reaching over 40 per cent of weekly income (Bradshaw and Morgan, 1987). Secondly, food is the item of household spending over which mothers are most likely to exercise direct control.

These two factors together mean that, while identified as a basic and essential resource, food is the area in which cutbacks are most often sought (Graham 1987b; Ritchie, 1990). In a recent

Table 8.1 Proportion of weekly income devoted to selected items of expenditure among two-parent households on benefit, Tyne and Wear.

	% of weekly spending
Basic necessities	
food	30
fuel	15
Other items	
clothes	8
tobacco	7
alcohol	4
transport	3

Source: Bradshaw and Holmes (1989), Table 5.13. (Reproduced by permission of the authors)

study of households with an unemployed head, there was virtually no change in the families' holdings of durable goods, such as televisions, during the early months of signing on. But their living standards deteriorated sharply for the majority of couples with children. Among those aged under 35, nearly half reported cutting back on food in the first three months after becoming unemployed (Heady and Smyth, 1989). Reflecting these financial pressures to economise through food, it is often in the diet they give their children that mothers experience most acutely what it means to be poor.

> As I see it, you get your bills in for a certain amount and you've got to pay it. You can't sort of say – well, I know some people do – but I can't say 'I won't pay that bill because I've got to buy some food'. I put away the money to pay that bill and if I haven't got anything left over to buy food with, then we have to manage.

> Food's the only place I find I can tighten up. The rest of it, they take it before you can get your hands on it really. So it's the food. The only place I can cut down is food. You've got to balance nutrition with a large amount of food which will keep them not hungry. I'd like to give them fresh fruit, whereas the good food has to be limited. Terrible, isn't it, when you think about it?[2]

Despite cutting back on food, low-income families consistently report that they run out of money before the end of the week. Expressed more formally, their weekly expenditure exceeds their weekly income (Berthoud and Kempson, 1992). A study of two-parent families on benefit found that the majority (58 per cent) spent more than their income, by an average of £21 a week (Bradshaw and Holmes, 1989). Spending more than you get means that living standards fall sharply through the week as first the money and then the food runs out.

> I get my money from my husband on dole day – Thursday. I do my big shopping that day at the supermarket. That's the day we have the best meal, usually with meat. From then on my main shopping is buying bread and milk at the local shop. By Monday or Tuesday, I'm out of money. Then I borrow maybe £10 from my sister – she can give it to me because she gets her money on a Tuesday. I pay back what I owe her on Thursday so she can keep going.[3]

> My biggest problem is providing food from Tuesday to Thursday. Look at my son there, he only has one pair of jeans. He had to wash them and dry them straight away and put them back on.[4]

Spending more than you have and borrowing to make it to the end of the week leaves many needs unmet. While the safety-net benefits, such as income support and unemployment benefit, are designed to provide for the basic needs of those without other sources of income, the evidence suggests that a significant proportion of claimant households are going short (Berthoud, 1989). Studies of living standards on benefit highlight the particular difficulties faced by one-parent and two-parent households with children: they consistently report more shortages of basic necessities, like clothes and shoes, and more unmet needs than other households. In a study by Bradshaw and Holmes of two-parent families on benefit, a considerable proportion of the weekly benefit went on paying for clothes, often through mail order catalogues and clothing clubs. Yet, three-quarters of the women and the men and 60 per cent of the children lacked more than two basic items of clothing. One in four families said that they were in desperate need of clothes and shoes (Bradshaw and Holmes, 1989).

A larger survey of households headed by unemployed people underlines the particular difficulties faced by young families with children in meeting basic needs (Heady and Smyth, 1989). The families were all two-parent families and, as Figure 8.4 suggests, they were more likely to report that they could not afford everything they needed than married couples without children. Among households with three or more dependent children

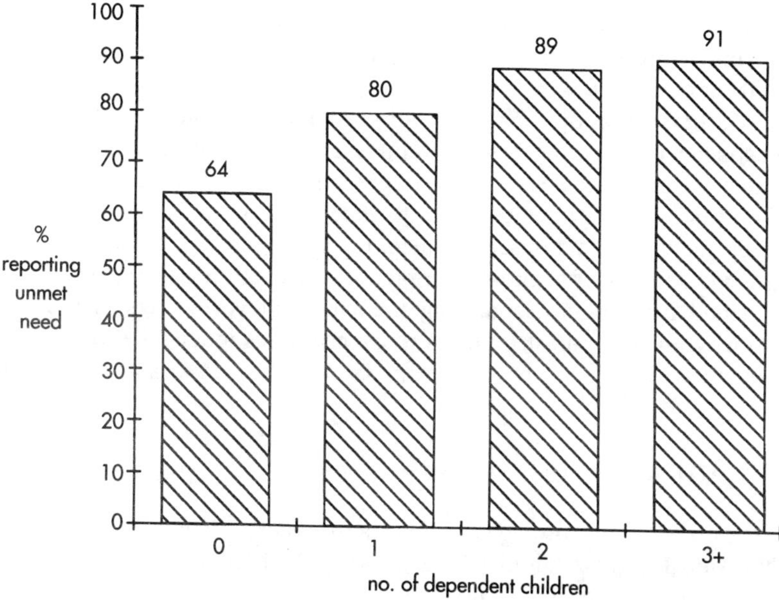

Figure 8.4 Unmet need reported by families of unemployed people who had signed on continuously for 15 months, married/cohabiting couples under 35.

Source: Heady and Smyth (1989), Volume I, derived from Table 9.4.

headed by an unemployed person under 35, over 90 per cent reported unmet needs.

Not having enough money for everyday needs has particular implications for those who are vested with the twin responsibilities of caring for health and making ends meet. It is often women who experience, in a particularly sharp and painful way, what it takes to survive on an income that threatens health. Some mothers live out this conflict without playing any direct role in the management of money. However, the evidence suggests that most women in low-income households are heavily involved in budgeting, taking more financial responsibility than those in better-off households (Pahl, 1989). In a study of 900 mothers in working class households, one in five of the mothers living with partners reported that they managed all the money and gave their partner his share. The proportion was higher (29 per cent) among those on income support than among those in households where earnings provided the major source of income (18 per cent) (Graham, 1992a).

Mothers develop a variety of strategies as they work to reconcile their caring responsibilities and their financial obligations. These strategies can be grouped under two broad headings. The first set of strategies seeks to meet health needs and make ends meet within household income. The second set looks to outside sources of support. In practice, these strategies are often pursued in tandem. Separating them out, however, signals the priority given by most mothers to managing as independently as possible.

8.4 Trying to survive without help

Women's labour provides a first and crucial defence against hardship for their families. Substituting their unpaid labour for money can help make up the shortfall between needs and resources. Women go to the launderette and wash clothes by hand when there is no washing machine; they walk to the supermarket, the antenatal clinic and the housing department when money must be saved on public and private transport. It is women, too, who often make more frequent trips to the shops when there is not enough cash or storage facilities to buy in bulk.

Paid work, too, provides a crucial strategy in the struggle to survive. As noted in Chapter 6, economic necessity is often the reason why women work – and return to work after they have children. Reflecting these financial pressures, women's earnings are typically devoted to essential items, like food and fuel, rent and childen's clothes, which play a direct part in protecting the health of their families.

Personal consumption provides a second area in which women (and their partners) can resist the impact of poverty on their children. Both historical and contemporary studies have recorded how women's living standards provide a buffer against poverty for other family members. Women deepen their own poverty by self-imposed cutbacks, taking their living standards further below what others would regard as a basic minimum. They cut out personal items and services: new clothes, shoes, underwear, make-up, hair-cuts and the use of public transport rarely appear on the expenditure diaries of mothers in low-income households (Bradshaw and Morgan, 1987; Bradshaw and Holmes, 1989). The picture that emerged in a 1990/1 study suggests that living on income support affects whether a mother usually has the money for her and her children's clothes in a very different way. While two-thirds of the mothers (66 per cent) felt that they usually had enough money for their children's clothes, the proportion fell by half, to one-third (33 per cent) when it came to their own clothes (Graham, 1992a).

> I'm a member of the Church Council and a governor of the (primary) School, those things I've kept up. I was on the PTA at St Joseph's (secondary school), I've dropped that. I did get to the point where I had no clothes to wear to go. . . . How could I go to those meetings with trainers with no soles and jeans with holes in? . . . I felt I could go to the primary school like that and they would understand, but not the secondary school, because the children are that much older. I don't think they would want me to turn up looking like that and I certainly wouldn't want to inflict it on them.[5]

However, cutting back on personal expenditure rarely produces the necessary economies. In such circumstances, mothers turn to a third strategy. They turn to collective items where they can restrict what they consume. A recurrent theme in studies of poverty is how mothers cut back on their own consumption of food in order to protect the living standards of children and partners. Mothers miss out meals and consume less to provide more for others.

> It's clear I'm sitting here for the children and it's for the children first. Whatever their important needs, that's what I try to fulfil. I give to them first and then myself. I can survive with eating or without eating or without new clothes but the children can't.[6]

An Irish survey points to the effects of cutting back on food on a mother's nutritional status (Lee and Gibney, 1989). The study was based in a large corporation housing estate that was chosen because it had high levels of unemployment and a population consisting mainly of families with young children. Three in four families were in receipt of welfare benefits. While diets were often poor among men and children, women always fared significantly worse in terms of nutrient intake. This comes across in the measures of recommended daily allowances (RDAs). RDAs are taken to represent the amount of each nutrient required to prevent deficiency rather than the amounts required for optimum health (Blackburn, 1991). Looking at vitamin C, the survey found that three times as many women as men were consuming less than 75 per cent of the RDA for vitamin C. With regard to iron intake, few problems were identified among the men in the sample. However, only half of the lone mothers achieved even half the RDA for iron. While mothers, and lone mothers in particular, were at greatest nutritional risk, the survey found no evidence that their children shared these nutritional disadvantages. Their diets were protected while their mothers' diets suffered. The patterns that lie behind the differences in nutritional status within families are graphically conveyed in the accounts that mothers have given of their lives.

> I'll cut down myself on food. Sometimes if we're running out the back end of the second week and there's not a lot for us to eat, I'll sort of give the kids it first and then see what's left. He (partner) is very good that way.[7]

> I buy half a pound of stewing meat of something and give that to Sid and the kiddies and then I just have the gravy – before I used to buy soya things and substitutes to meat but I can't afford that now.[8]

The 'individualising' of the family's lifestyle is apparent, too, in other areas of consumption, including clothes, fuel and transport. Mothers describe how they set different standards of dress for themselves and their children, standards matched by their more economical use of heating in the home. For example, a mother in a study of families facing unemployment noted that the cost of fuel meant that she did not light the fire during the day when her children were at school, but saved the limited fuel supplies to protect their standard of living. As she put it, 'as long as it's warm when the children get home, I'm not bothered about myself' (Ritchie, 1990, p.36).

> I'll go to jumble sales for my clothes, I won't go to a catalogue for mine. But I'm not seeing me kid and me husband walk to town in second-hand clothes. I'll make do for myself but I won't make do for them.[9]

> I put the central heating on for one hour before the kids go to bed and one hour before they get up. I sit in a sleeping bag once they've gone to bed.

> When the children are in bed, I turn the heating off and use a blanket or an extra cardigan.[10]

These personal cost-cutting measures are mediated through the wider household distribution of resources. In many low-income households, women are supported by their partners, with both parents cutting back to protect the living standards of their children (Ritchie, 1990).

> Now and again we get something out of a catalogue, you know, because with two kids you've mainly got to keep them clothed. . . . I go to jumble sales. . . . Now the jacket I've got on now, I got that for £2 off a lass down the road you know, she's a friend of the wife's who's split with her husband and asked if I wanted to buy a jacket. I say 'yeah' because I could do with one, you know, warm jacket, that's the only jacket I've really got that's decent.[11]

In other families, partners' control of resources may constrain women's attempts to look after health within the limits of the resources available to her. Carefully worked out strategies may flounder because of the lifestyles pursued by others. For example, women have described how it is difficult to cut down on food when cooking for a partner who expects meat at his main meal (Charles and Kerr, 1988). Partner's preferences can also make it more difficult to control household fuel consumption and transport costs, and to effect cutbacks in personal consumption.

> I don't cut back on food. I mean my husband likes his joint of meat once a week and that's it.

> I don't spend any money on make-up or clothes for myself, so I can't save on that. I can't really give up on any social life, in going out or anything, because we don't really have one. I'd get rid of the car but it's his car, as he says, and I don't think he'd be prepared to sell it unless we got into real financial difficulties. I don't drive. I walk everywhere.

> I turn it off when I'm in on my own and put a blanket on myself. Sometimes we both do in the evening but my husband doesn't like being cold and puts the heating back on.[12]

With or without a supportive partner, managing independently remains a common goal for many mothers as they search for ways of meeting health needs while cutting back on health resources. However, as described in Chapter 7, increasing dependency on others is a reality for many families on low incomes.

8.5 Relying on others

For mothers faced with the task of reconciling an inadequate income with the health-needs of families, small additional sources of income can make a significant difference to living standards. The major source of independent income, and one paid direct to mothers, is child benefit. As noted in Chapter 7, it reaches almost all eligible White, Asian and African–Caribbean mothers. While its value fell in real terms through the 1980s, the evidence suggests that it forms an integral and essential part of mothers' budgeting and caring strategies. Mothers in low-income households typically receive their benefit weekly while mothers in better-off households are more likely to have the benefit paid on a monthly basis into their bank account (Graham, 1987b). Like their earnings from paid work, mothers spend their child benefit on items related to housekeeping and childcare: on food, children's clothes and shoes, and school expenses (Walsh and Lister, 1985).

For those struggling to make ends meet, child benefit can provide a vital mid-week stop-gap, tiding mothers over until their major source of income, in the form of earnings, income support or a housekeeping allowance, arrives.

> The housekeeping money is just about enough. I've got it now that I budget myself with the housekeeping until Monday or Tuesday when I get my child benefit. That's what budgeting is all about. It's got to last but I never have a penny left by Tuesday morning.[13]

As a universal benefit, child benefit supports mothers in households with incomes which, while modest, are above the threshold for means-tested benefits (Walsh and Lister, 1985). It reaches, too, mothers trapped in hidden poverty in better-off households. As a benefit paid direct to mothers, it can provide a lifeline for women in relationships where they are denied access to the income they need to care for themselves and their children.

> I know there is also an argument that well-off families shouldn't get the benefit, but the problem is where to draw the line. We are just the wrong side of the line usually drawn for help, and certainly wouldn't want to do without child benefit, indeed we would find it very difficult.[14]

> I spend my child benefit on children's clothes, if they need them, and also things for the house. I look on it as housekeeping money, children's clothes money, my money. He doesn't have it to spend on him. I have it to spend on us.[15]

Beyond this universal benefit lie the discretionary sources of support. Chapter 7 described how low-income households are increasingly dependent on credit and burdened by debt. Multiple credit and debt commitments are common, with families working to pay off loans on incomes which are already insufficient to cover household costs and day-to-day expenses. One case study, provided by Berthoud and Kempson in their study of credit and debt gives a sense of what 'multiple debt' means in everyday terms for families on low incomes.

> A married couple with four children: one of school age, one working and two unemployed. The parents' income was £91.25 a week (£84 income support and £7.25 child benefit), plus full housing benefit. The older children contributed £10 a week each to the housekeeping. The couple had the following credit commitments:
>
> - One HP agreement: £480 for a washing machine, paid back through their electric slot meter.
> - three outstanding loans from a check company, one of £300 and two at £100 taken out to buy clothes and to pay bills, with repayments of £26 a week.
> - a social fund loan of £190 to meet the costs of decorating, with repayments deducted from their income support at source.
> - a £382 loan from a finance house for a carpet, being repaid at £14 a month.
> - repayments of £15 a week to a mail-order catalogue for clothing.
> - a loan of £40 from the wife's mother.[16]

Studies have highlighted the importance of relatives and friends as a source of mutual support when times are tough. Mutual support systems are typically mediated through women.

reflecting and reinforcing the gendered organisation of care within families. Thus, most of the day-to-day help received by mothers comes from other women, and from female friends and relatives in particular (Graham, 1986; Wilmott, 1987). Their mothers and their partners' mothers play an especially important part in this informal economy of care, providing practical help with childcare and giving material support, typically in kind rather than cash. They give food to their daughters and search out clothes for grandchildren.

For mothers struggling to meet their health-keeping and housekeeping responsibilities, such gifts help to protect the living standards of their children (Craig and Glendinning, 1990; Ritchie, 1990). Gifts can become regularised, with grandmothers and great-grandmothers becoming the main providers of children's clothes and shoes.

> My mum is always buying things. If she sees a nice dress for her, she'll buy it. A couple of times she's sent money for Easter eggs and school photos. Occasionally, she's given me £5 or £10 if I go down to see her and says 'treat yourself and don't tell Dave, treat yourself'.[17]

Material support can be more deeply woven into women's budgeting strategies, providing essential health resources, like food, both on a routine basis and in times of crisis.

> We have three good meals at my mum's, Saturday, Sunday and Monday, and we always have meat and fresh vegetables then. It would worry me if I was having to feed her all the time but knowing that three days out of seven she's getting good meals, it doesn't worry me so much. And more often than not, when I come back from me mum's, I find little bits in the bottom of the bag because she feels sorry for us.

> If I've had a big bill, occasionally I've had to say to my mum, 'I've no money left, can I come down for the week?' and I've had to go down there. Somehow or other I manage to get through and I think it's because my parents help me.[18]

While parents provide a lifeline for many women in poverty, they are not always an unproblematic source of help (see Chapter 7). Women may not have access to relatives who are able or willing to respond. The restrictions governing immigration can leave Asian claimants without parents in the United Kingdom. The poverty of family members and their attitudes to kin-support, too, can limit what they can provide. In a study of the households of redundant steelworkers, kin were providing extra help – mostly in the form of food and clothes for the children – for less than a third of the families (Morris, 1983).

Further, asking relatives for money and other forms of material help may undermine the moral base on which relations with kin are built. Asking for help transgresses the ethic of independence which governs many families and has been strongly articulated by Asian parents on benefit (Sadiq-Sangster, 1991). Further, loans and gifts of money from relatives can run counter to the expected patterns of support. As one White single mother noted about the financial support she was receiving from her mother, 'it's not very nice doing it because I feel I should be helping her' (Cohen, 1991b, p.40).

> This is the first time in my working life I have to go to the family to ask them for money. I've never asked them for anything before . . . then all of a sudden, you become partly dependent on them. . . . It's very difficult.[19]

Receiving such help can knock on already fragile self-esteem. It can also leave a lingering anxiety that relatives may call in their loan at any time: an anxiety that ran through the accounts of Asian parents on benefit in one recent study (Sadiq-Sangster, 1991).

> Whenever they want it, they can ask for it any time, even today, they could say they want it back. . . . Now I'm ever so depressed. I think how am I ever going to pay it all back. All day and night it's on my mind, honestly, I can't sleep at night for thinking about this loan.[20]

In exploring how mothers work to make ends meet, this chapter has drawn a distinction between strategies which involve surviving independently and those that involve outsiders in the financial affairs of the family. Mothers rarely have an option on which set of approaches to use. Instead, they typically survive from day to day by combining strategies and juggling money between the pressing and competing demands on their limited income.

I've got £24.44 to pay for the rent, I have the electricity bill to pay – I have just paid £20 off that – I've got a £53 gas bill and now he needs trousers. So I've got to juggle it around: he's got to have trousers or he can't go to school. So one bill has to wait, so it will have to be the gas bill, because the rent has got to be paid. This is it, this is how you go, you just juggle it around.[21]

Notes

1. Parents quoted in Cohen (1991b), p.28.
2. Two lone mothers on benefit, quoted in Graham (1992b), pp.218–19.
3. Mother quoted in Daly (1989), p.31.
4. Mother quoted in Daly (1988), p.81.
5. Lone mother on income support quoted in Cohen (1991c), p.5.
6. Parent quoted in Sadiq-Sangster (1991), p.3.
7. Mother on benefit quoted in Graham (1985), p.144.
8. Mother on benefit quoted in Ritchie (1990), p.35.
9. Mother on benefit quoted in Craig and Glendinning (1990), p.31.
10. Mothers on benefit quoted in Graham (1985), p.246.
11. Unemployed married father quoted in Ritchie (1990), p.36.
12. Three mothers in low-income households, unpublished data from Graham (1985).
13. Mother in non-claimant household quoted in Graham (1985), p.91.
14. Mother quoted in Walsh and Lister (1985), p.6.
15. Married mother quoted in Graham (1985), p.93.
16. Taken from case study given in Berthoud and Kempson (1992), p.107.
17. Mother on benefit quoted in Graham (1992b), p.221.
18. Ibid., pp.221–2.
19. Parent on income support quoted in Cohen (1991b), p.40.
20. Asian mother on income support who had borrowed £500 from her husband's relatives quoted in Sadiq-Sangster (1991), p.4.
21. Lone mother quoted in Cohen (1991b), p.31.

CHAPTER 9

KEEPING GOING

9.1 Introduction

In the course of this book, women have provided their own record of what it costs to care for health in circumstances of hardship. However, as with other dimensions of their lives, women's accounts of their health carry little scientific weight. They are seen to provide a less reliable guide to their experiences than the information gathered through the formal data collection agencies. It is through government statistics and social surveys that the official picture of women's health has been constructed.

The two sections below outline aspects of this picture, pointing to data which confirm that ill-health among mothers is linked to heavy caring responsibilities and restricted access to material resources. The third and fourth sections of the chapter examine how mothers work to keep on caring in these circumstances. They focus on cigarette smoking as a routine and a resource used by a large majority of White mothers caring for children in low-income households.

9.2 Gender differences in health

In Britain, as in other industrialised countries, there are systematic differences in the health experiences of men and women. Women suffer more ill-health than men but live longer. Men are more likely to die prematurely and to suffer more life-threatening illnesses while women experience more physical illness and disability across their longer lifespan (Blaxter, 1990; Devis, 1990; Bebbington, 1991). The evidence suggests that women also have poorer psychosocial health, see their GPs more often for mental health problems and are more frequently prescribed psychotropic drugs for anxiety and depression (N. Wells, 1987; Office of Population Censuses and Surveys, 1990b). As Jennie Popay and Mel Bartley put it, 'whilst women get the quantity of life years, men get the quality' (Popay and Bartley, 1989, p.89).

A variety of explanations have been put forward to explain this gender difference in health. Biological differences between men and women, particularly those relating to pregnancy and childbirth, explain part of the difference. But other factors are clearly at work. One influential set of perspectives suggests that the higher rates of morbidity among women reflect their greater willingness to report symptoms and to act on them. The suggested reason for their greater propensity to feel ill is that their domestic responsibilities give them more opportunity to take on a sick role (Verbrugge, 1985). In other words, women are not 'really' more unwell and unhappy than men: it is their role as women which allows them to express how they feel.

Feminist researchers, however, have challenged this view. They suggest that women's greater reported morbidity is not an artefact of differential illness behaviour but, instead, reflects real differences in the health experiences of men and women. Women are more unwell and unhappy than men because of the work they do and the conditions in which they do it (Popay and Bartley, 1989; Payne, 1991). Evidence on class differences in women's health lends support to this kind of perspective, pointing to the way in which their health is related to the material circumstances in which they live. Women married to men at the bottom of the class hierarchy report more physical symptoms and long-term illnesses than women married to men higher up the social class scale (Blaxter, 1990; Office of Population Censuses and Surveys, 1991a). They are also more likely to report feelings of anxiety, depression and stress which suggest that their emotional health is poor (Blaxter, 1990). Reflecting their higher levels of emotional distress, women assigned to social classes IV and V are more likely to consult a GP about a mental health problem than women in social classes I and II (Office of Population Censuses and Surveys, 1990b).

While 'race' tends to be left out of analyses of health

inequalities, the limited evidence supports a perspective that links women's health to the social conditions in which they live and work. As Chapters 2 and 6 noted, Black women are clustered in manual working class households and in the lower paid sectors of the economy. Further, Black women have described how racism as well as economic hardship runs through their everyday lives (Bryan *et al.*, 1985; Mama, 1989). While racism is bound into how Black people experience their health, studies suggest that it is not part of the way White people understand health in Britain (Eyles and Donovan, 1990).

> (Racism) is there and you know it's there. You can feel it all the time, everywhere. You know you're black.
>
> I don't even like to think what the effect is. It can wear people down. It makes you feel bad inside, angry, and then one day it will come out. This racial thing, we will get over it. We have to live through it and be strong. We have to. It's the only way to carry on, to survive.[1]

While there is now a considerable body of research which points to the way in which social divisions impact on women's health, relatively little of it focuses on women with children. The section below examines some of this research and the light it sheds on how the everyday lives of mothers are etched into their sense of physical and emotional well-being.

9.3 The health of mothers

Secondary analyses of large scale surveys such as the General Household Survey and the Health and Lifestyle Survey suggest that the broad gender differences in health are reproduced in the patterns of health among parents. Mothers are more likely to report recent illnesses than fathers and are less likely to rate their health as good (Popay and Jones, 1990).

> I was really tired – normally I can wake, feed him and go back – but this night I just couldn't wake up. And he was crying and I'd fed him and he still wasn't settling – this was when I was breast feeding him and he wasn't getting enough . . . I changed him and fed him the bottle and he still wouldn't go back. And I went to get another nappy 'cos he'd wet again. And I just went and sat down

with my head in the airing cupboard and I just started to cry, 'Oh for God's sake, shut up!'. That was just that night. It was just being tired. If I can get my sleep, I can cope with it.[2]

Tiredness seems to be a side-effect of parenthood that is particularly linked to being a mother. Analysing data from the Health and Lifestyle Survey, Popay found that women with children were more likely to report always feeling tired than men with children. Among mothers, tiredness appeared to be linked to additional caring responsibilities: to having younger children and to having more children. As Table 9.1 suggests, the proportions reporting that they always felt tired were higher among women with children under one year and among women with three or more children than among women with older and fewer children. Among men, this upward trend in tiredness was more muted (Table 9.1).

A similar gender difference emerges when parents with disabled children are looked at separately. In the OPCS surveys of disability, over one in three (37 per cent) married mothers felt that having a disabled child had had an effect on their health. In contrast, only one in eight (13 per cent) felt that their husband's health had been affected. The most common health problems reported by the mothers were anxiety and depression, and tiredness and exhaustion (Meltzer *et al.*, 1989).

Table 9.1 Proportion of mothers and fathers aged 18–39 reporting always feeling tired by age and number of children.

	Women (%)	Men (%)
Age of youngest child		
under 1 year	39	20
1–5 years	38	23
6–16 years	31	20
Number of children		
1 child	32	20
2 children	34	22
3 or more children	36	22

Source: Data from Health and Lifestyle Survey analysed in Popay (1992), p.106, Table 6.1.

The accounts included in earlier parts of the book suggest that mothers try to ignore their tiredness, like the other symptoms they experience, in order to keep going. Mothers are frequently aware of this accommodation, recognising that their caring responsibilities leave them little time to be ill (Pill and Stott, 1982; Cornwell, 1984). As mothers have repeatedly pointed out to researchers, their caring responsibilities can blunt their sensitivity to their own needs. Rather than making it easier to be ill, they have described how caring for others can make it harder to take sick leave from domestic life.

> I would never stay in bed unless like, I mean, I was being sick . . . that's the only reason. . . . I still have to look after the children . . . lying in bed I just find I worry and I tend to think, 'Oh my goodness, what was that noise, I'd better deal with it'. The men are fine, they're just lucky that they can switch off and it's probably a better thing. . . . We're all – women – like that.[3]

> We have the heavy tasks. We rush to get everyone to work, we rush to work, rush at work. Then you come home, you've got the washin' or cooking or ironing. It's never ending. Time you finished, you have to get to bed. . . . Then you get a few hours' rest before you gotta be up again for work. . . . Tiredness can wear you down.[4]

Mothers' accounts record how the circumstances as well as the responsibilities of caring affect how they feel about themselves. In previous chapters, mothers have described the toll that caring for children takes on their health when family lives are disrupted by homelessness and the search for decent accommodation. In the last two chapters, women spoke of the additional burdens of caring when money is short, struggling with the stigma, stress and the sacrifices involved in trying to meet health needs and manage debts at the same time.

> The kids might be looking for money to go somewhere and do you know what I would do? I would scream at them and throw the loan books at them and say: 'Where do you think I'm going to get the money?' My 13 year old son was so concerned that he asked me could we sit down and talk about it. I just snapped at him to mind his own business. I think I went through a nervous breakdown without realising it.[5]

The links between mothers' lives and mothers' health are

captured more clinically in survey data. Figure 9.1 is based on an analysis of General Household Survey data and focuses on married and cohabiting women (Popay and Jones, 1990). It takes three measures of health: long-standing illness, recent illness and a self-assessment of whether health has been generally good over the past twelve months. Recognising the problems associated with the traditional measures of women's class position, the researchers identified three broad 'standard of living' groups. Women were allocated to one of the groups on the basis of their housing tenure and, for council tenants, on whether the household was in receipt of selected means-tested benefits which provided an approximate income line. Using these three standard-of-living groups, Popay and Jones found an inverse relationship between the health of married mothers and the socioeconomic status of their household. One fifth (22 per cent) of the mothers living in owner-occupied homes reported a long-standing illness: among the mothers in council-owned homes and receiving benefits, the proportion was one in three (34 per cent). Similarly, while over 70 per cent of mothers in the highest standard-of-living group reported that their health had been generally good over the past year, the proportion fell to just over a half among mothers in the poorest circumstances (see Figure 9.1).

Other surveys confirm the patterns of health among married and cohabiting mothers summarised in Figure 9.1. In the national Health and Lifestyle Survey, for example, working class mothers who were living with men described more physical symptoms of ill-health and more long term illnesses and disabilities than middle class mothers who lived with men (Blaxter, 1990). They also reported more emotional health problems, like anxiety and difficulty sleeping.

> As soon as the bills come my blood pressure's up. . . . As soon as it comes through the letterbox . . . and sometimes I can't open it then and there because I just haven't the strength, the emotional strength, to open it and see what the amount is. I have to put the letter up and wait until I feel mentally I can face looking at it.[6]

The experiences of lone mothers provide further evidence that both the responsibilities and the circumstances of caring play an important part in women's health. Analyses of GHS data suggest that lone mothers report poorer health than mothers in two-parent households (Popay and Jones, 1990). They are more likely to have both long-standing and recent illnesses, and are less likely to assess their health over the last twelve months as good (Figure 9.2).

> I find I get a lot of headaches and it's all down to stress. It's the situation I'm in. . . . I mean it's the money and the situation that everything is my responsibility, you know. I never go out, never get time to relax. . . . I think it's stress (that causes) headaches, high blood pressure, all this. . . .[7]

Among lone mothers, as among married and cohabiting mothers, material circumstances are closely linked to health status. Figure 9.3 suggests that lone mothers in owner-occupied housing are less likely to report long-standing and recent illnesses than lone mothers who are council tenants, but are not dependent on the main means-tested benefits. Lone mothers who are both tenants and claimants have the worst health profile of the three groups. In this group, less than half (43 per cent)

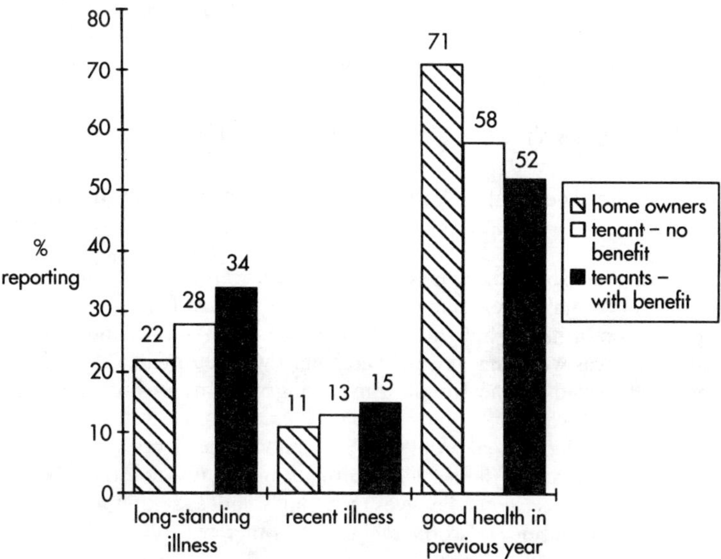

Figure 9.1 Health of married/cohabiting mothers by housing tenure and income.

Source: Data from the General Household Survey 1980–2 analysed in Popay and Jones (1990), p. 517, derived from Table 5.

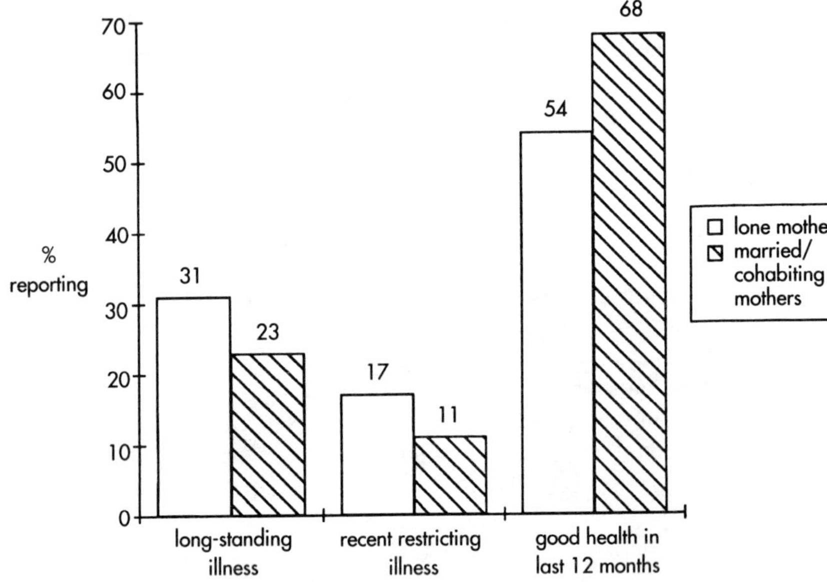

Figure 9.2 Health of lone mothers and married/cohabiting mothers.

Source: Data from the General Household Survey 1980–2 analysed in Popay and Jones (1990), p. 510, derived from Table 1.

describe their general health as good and nearly four in ten (39 per cent) report a long-standing illness (Popay and Jones, 1990).

> It's various stresses, you know, little bits and pieces all put together to make a big one. My money worries. At first, it used to get on top of me. I thought I can't live like this. And I found even though I was worrying, it wasn't helping. I was getting in a state. It was silly. And all the trouble I'm having with my ex-husband. I never know when he's going to 'phone up to say he wants to see the children, that's a problem. You know, the access visits. I agreed he could see them once a fortnight but he just doesn't come and when he does come he gives me a day's notice. I don't want to upset the children. I'd sooner him not bother with the children. But there's another worry.[8]

The way in which heavy caring responsibilities and poor material circumstances combine to undermine women's health is perhaps most powerfully conveyed by mothers living in temporary accommodation. Something of their health experiences

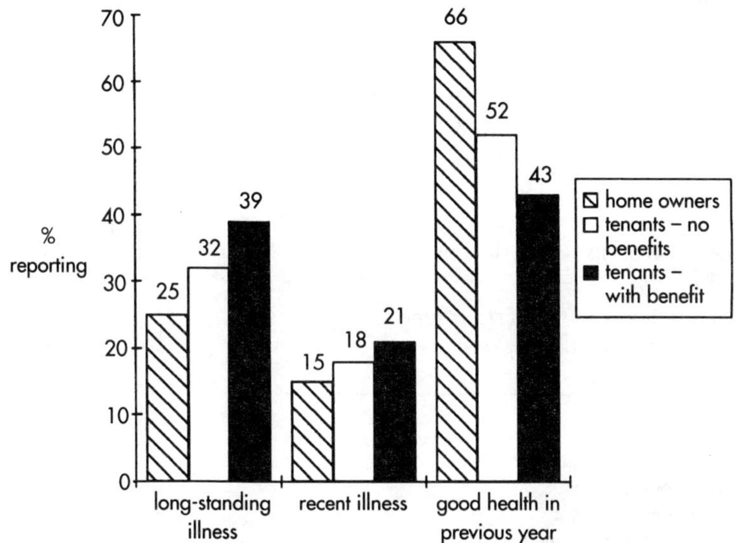

Figure 9.3 Health of lone mothers by housing tenure and income.

Source: Data from the General Household Survey 1980–2 analysed in Popay and Jones (1990), p. 517, derived from Table 5.

was conveyed in Chapter 3. Caring for children in cramped, unsanitary and insecure conditions, and with little time or space for yourself is reflected in high levels of physical illness and emotional distress.

> I've never had a health visitor since the baby's been born. I can't get registered with a doctor. I've lived here a year without one, and with a baby. He's been in hospital twice. He caught a virus from the hotel which was growing in his bowel. He lost over six pound in a week. Then he had a blocked intestine so he was in hospital for nearly two weeks that time. . . . I feel so old, I mean I don't class myself as being young. I'm 34. But I don't know – I feel so old now, so very, very old.

> Being homeless is terrible, it's – being less of everything. I was in the hotel seven months; to me it was seven million years. When they told me I had a flat, I nearly fainted! I jumped! When I came and saw this place, I didn't want to come. But then again I had to come because they said, 'you've only got one choice'. If I had said

> no, they would have made me wait another year. I couldn't do that, I would have gone mental there.[9]

In one survey of 56 women and their children living in bed and breakfast hostels, mothers described how they felt generally run down and tired, and were particularly susceptible to coughs and colds. The majority (61 per cent) reported regular headaches and migraines (Conway, 1988). Nearly four in five reported being unhappy most of the time. Over three in five described themselves as often losing their temper (Table 9.2).

Table 9.2 Symptoms of stress reported by 56 mothers in bed and breakfast accommodation.

	%
Unhappy most of the time	79
Tired most of the time	73
Often lose my temper	63
Often can't sleep at night	61
The children get on top of me	59
Burst into tears for no reason	43

Source: Conway (1988), derived from Table 3.1.

The experiences of mothers in temporary accommodation capture, in stark relief, how women's health and conditions are linked. They underline how heavy caring responsibilities and limited material resources leave mothers with chronic health problems: with repeated headaches and feeling unhappy and tired most of the time. The next two sections explore how mothers keep going when poor health is an integral part of their experience of caring in hardship.

9.4 Getting through

Most mothers care for their children single-handed, and at times and in places where there may be no other adults present. For many mothers, the places in which they care are less than health-promoting. Shortage of money brings additional anxieties and makes it hard to escape from either home or neighbourhood, or to access resources which could give solace and strength to mothers who know their health is giving way.

> It's hard to explain. I feel that everything in life is on a downward spiral at the moment, I can't see anything to be really hopeful about. . . . I used to have dreams about the future; I don't care to think about the future too much. I still try to hope.[10]

As mothers try to hope, they also find ways to keeping going. They develop routines and resources which help them face each day and survive it. To be effective, these routines and resources need to be part of daily domestic life, easily accessed and used by mothers as they go about the business of caring. They must enable mothers both to maintain their health-keeping and housekeeping responsibilities and to find some respite from them.

A number of routines and resources meet these exacting criteria. Women have spoken, for example, of how relationships with partners, parents and friends can provide both ongoing support and a time-out for relaxing and refuelling.

> When I get het up I go upstairs and sit down and do a lot of deep thinking and I usually find it's something you have to cope with. I often talk things out with my boyfriend. I find just opening up and telling him what I feel often helps. But it's often too trivial things to actually talk about it.

> Well I just think 'I know I'm not going to starve, and the rent's paid so there's a roof over my head so everything else they'll just have to sing for. They'll just have to wait'. I've got like that now. And I know if things do get too bad, I can go down to mum and dad's. I think it does help having so many people around me. I think if I had no friends and my family lived a way off and I was stuck in this house every day with Michele, I'd go out of my mind. But I think it's just mind over matter really, you just get on and do it. You either cope or you don't, when it gets down to it.[11]

Hobbies such as listening to music and watching television can serve as a safety-valve when the pressure builds up and as leisure activities through which to unwind. When children are occupied, are out or are asleep, the opportunities increase, with greater scope for leisure and work activities (including paid work) to provide a time-out from caring.

> My most relaxing thing is a nice, hot, soapy bubbly bath, with a book. A cup of coffee to take up. That's a luxury for me, to lie and soak in the bath for an hour or so, that's lovely.

> I just sit and watch TV or listen to music or just sit and think. I'm

> a Christian and I tend to just delve into my faith. That helps tremendously.[12]

For some mothers, religious beliefs and rituals can be an important source of solace, giving a peace of mind and an inner strength when times are tough. Faith has been highlighted as a resource in studies in which Asian and African–Caribbean women have spoken about their daily lives (Gabe and Thorogood, 1986; Eyles and Donovan, 1990).

> I never cry, just call on Him, because He is there to help me in all my needs. I have faith in God. I don't take tablets. God is always there with me, to heal.

> Prayer helps very much, even when you are very depressed. It would help me more than the tranquillisers. . . . Those who believe in God and pray to God, they must be certainly healthier than the others, mentally and physically.

> You should be able to talk to Him all the time. It doesn't matter where you are. . . . If you've got problems, you should talk to Him about it. He is the Great Psychiatrist.[13]

As the accounts given above suggest, tranquillisers provide another way of finding relief from the pressures of everyday life. However, women tend to be deeply ambivalent about taking psychotropic drugs like the benzodiazepine compounds, which include valium, librium and ativan. They are aware that these drugs provide on-the-spot relief, with the properties of the drugs well adapted to the particular strains that go with caring. But women express concerns about long-term dependency and the health-costs of repeated use (Gabe and Thorogood, 1986).

> I hate the stuff, I detest the stuff. You know you've taken a drug when you've taken valium. But I can't say I can do without them. I don't want to break right down because I won't be able to pick up the pieces. I'd rather stay the way I am.[14]

Like psychotropic drugs, other coping strategies can have contradictory effects, helping women care but bringing potential risks to health. Giving children sweets is seen as a major cause of tooth decay and one that instils bad dental health habits. However, sweets can help keep the peace in situations of stress. They can be used to encourage good behaviour; instantly provided at crisis points on buses and in the street, and held out as a reward in the home (Kerr and Charles, 1983). Cigarette smoking is another example of a habit which promotes and undermines well-being at the same time. It has been identified as the single most significant cause of ill-health and premature death in Britain, and one that can be linked directly to the behaviour of individuals. For the 29 per cent of women who smoke in Britain, 'giving up is the single most important step they could take to improve their health' (Department of Health, 1989).

Giving up smoking is seen as a particularly important step for pregnant women and women with young children. Smoking in pregnancy has been associated with an increased risk of miscarriage, low birth weight and raised perinatal mortality, while maternal smoking after birth has been related to lower height in primary school children and to increased risk of respiratory complaints (Department of Health, 1989). At over £2 a pack, cigarette smoking is clearly a coping strategy with financial as well as health costs. As a result, it tends to be seen as an irresponsible indulgence, a pattern of behaviour which suggests to those on the outside of family life that mothers are neither as caring nor as poor as they claim.

9.5 Cigarette smoking

In the 1950s, cigarette smoking was a habit with no clear class identity. Four in ten women in all social classes were smokers (Graham, 1988a). Since then, the class profile of cigarette smoking has shifted markedly. While smoking prevalence has declined among women in all social classes, it has declined more rapidly among those in higher socioeconomic groups. Today, cigarette smoking – like deaths from coronary heart disease and lung cancer – is strongly, and increasingly, class related (Pugh *et al.*, 1991). The General Household Survey suggests that 16 per cent of women classified as members of professional households are cigarette smokers; among women in unskilled manual households, the proportion is 36 per cent (Office of Population Censuses and Surveys, 1991d).

National data highlight, too, that it is White women who make up most of Britain's female smokers (Graham, 1988a). Among

White women, it is those engaged in activities traditionally assigned to women who appear particularly likely to smoke. Thus, women who are not in paid work and who are caring for children have higher smoking prevalence rates than women in employment and those without children. Figure 9.4 conveys something of the scale of difference among married women in the 16 to 24 and 25 to 34 age groups who live with and without children under 16. It suggests that among women aged 25 to 34 without dependent children, less than a quarter (23 per cent) are cigarette smokers. Among women aged 16 to 24 with children, the proportion is twice as high. Among this group, half (51 per cent) are smokers.

When caring responsibilities combine with poor material circumstances, cigarette smoking shifts more sharply from a minority into a majority habit. In a recent study of 900 mothers caring for young children in manual working-class households, 68 per cent of those dependent on income support were cigarette smokers (Graham, 1992a). Other studies have uncovered simi-

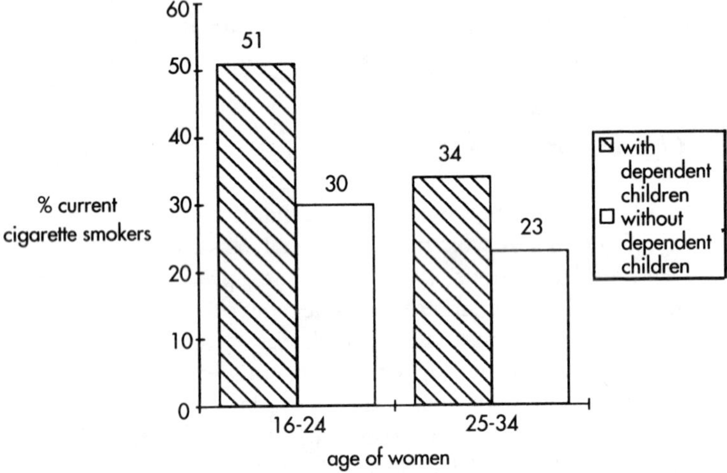

Figure 9.4 Cigarette smoking among married/cohabiting women with and without dependent children, Britain, 1988.

Note: Dependent children are persons under 16 or aged 16 to 18 and in full-time education, in the family unit and living in the household.
Source: Office of Population Censuses and Surveys (1990a), derived from Table 5.14(b).

larly high smoking prevalence rates. In a study of households with children in Edinburgh, Glasgow and London, nearly 60 per cent of the households had no one in paid employment and two-thirds of the homes were damp. The proportion of women who smoked was 70 per cent (Hunt *et al.*, 1988). Smoking prevalence among men who live their lives under the shadow of poverty and unemployment is also high (Ginnety, 1985).

High smoking prevalence is reflected in high levels of spending on tobacco in low-income households. The budgeting strategies outlined in Chapter 8 suggest that, as a non-essential personal item, parents would spend little on tobacco, saving their money for collective necessities like food and fuel. However, low-income households spend more not less on tobacco than better-off households (Central Statistical Office, 1991). Like food and fuel, spending on tobacco is inversely related to income: more is spent proportionately on tobacco as household income falls. More is also spent in absolute terms in lower income households. While many would regard it as a luxury item, tobacco spending has the hallmark of a necessity: something that mothers describe spending more on when they have less to spend.

> I try to cut down to save money but cigarettes are my one luxury and at the moment they feel a bit like a necessity.[15]

> Eventually, I'd like to give up smoking but with the divorce and everything, I don't think I can at the moment. It's all I've got for myself.[16]

Qualitative studies of women's smoking suggest that tobacco is a necessity as well as a luxury because smoking helps mothers with heavy caring responsibilities keep going when their personal and material resources are overstretched (Graham, 1987c; J. Wells, 1987). In one study of mothers with preschool children, women described how smoking was part of a daily routine, marking, along with a cup of tea or coffee, the spaces of time snatched from the demanding schedule of caring for children. Their children were still with them and often still demanding, but a cigarette and a cup of coffee provided a time-out, a moment to rest and refuel. As one mother put it, 'When I've finished something, I always sit down and have a cigarette' (Graham, 1988a, p.379). Other women similarly described how smoking was part of the way they cared, and kept on caring.

> I smoke when I'm sitting down, having a cup of coffee. It's part and parcel of resting. Definitely, because it doesn't bother me if I haven't got a cigarette when I'm working. If I can keep working, doing the housework and the washing and the ironing and things like that, and I'm busy, I won't bother smoking but if I'm sitting down chatting or sitting having a cup of coffee, then I smoke. If I'm busy, it doesn't bother me, but it's nice to sit down afterwards and have a cigarette.[17]

> When they are all screaming and fighting in here and in the kitchen, I'm ready to blow up so I just light up a cigarette. It calms me down when I'm under so much stress.[18]

As the second account above indicates, cigarettes are associated not only with the maintenance of normal caring routines. They are also part of the way women cope with breakdowns in these patterns of caring. When faced with demands they cannot meet, mothers have described how they create a space – symbolic if not real – between them and their children and fill this space with a self-directed activity (Graham, 1988a). Smoking a cigarette provides a self-directed activity which can be instantly accessed when mothers feel that their breaking point has been reached.

> Sometimes I put him outside the room, shut the door and put the radio on full blast and I've sat down and had a cigarette, calmed down and fetched him in again.[19]

> I send them up to their bedroom when they're getting too much for me. When I see the danger signs looming, I think they're best out of the way. I sit down and have a cigarette and a cup of tea. After 10 minutes, I feel guilty and call them down. Usually the crisis has passed by then.[20]

Viewed within the context of mothers' daily lives, cigarette smoking appears to be a way of meeting rather than shirking responsibility. It provides a way of coping with the constant and unremitting demands of caring: a way of temporarily escaping without leaving the room. Cigarettes appear to be particularly finely tuned to caring in hardship, enabling mothers to remain calm in a situation where resources are few and responsibilities are many. Smoking offers an escape – however temporary and artificial – from the grind of cutting back and making do. Male partners can escape in other ways: for women, however, cigarettes may provide the only moment when poverty can be suspended and they can join a world of personal consumption that most people take for granted. They can become members of a society where small luxuries, small indulgences, are an everyday experience.

> I couldn't face a day without cigarettes. That's all we've got now.
>
> My husband goes out three times a week drinking with his mates. I don't go. Smoking is my form of relaxation . . .
>
> My boyfriend has his pleasure. He drinks. The only pleasure I have is smoking.
>
> It's the only thing I do myself, isn't it? I have to do things for the baby and for my husband, but smoking is about the only thing I can do for myself.[21]

Mothers describe the place of sweets in the lives of their children in similar ways. While damaging to their health, they provide one small area of consumption where their children's lifestyles converge with those of their peers.

> If we afford it, we do like to get them a lolly when the (ice cream) van comes round because all the kids are out there. The first week (after the fortnightly payment of benefit) and going into the second, they can have a lolly. But after that, we haven't got much money left so we can't let them have it.
>
> I feel I have to give them sweets sometimes as they don't get toys and clothes. They won't ever get new toys or new clothes, but I can afford 10p for them to buy sweets.[22]

Yet, such resources offer a very contradictory kind of support. They help and hurt mothers and children at the same time. Although health-sustaining, personal coping strategies are often also health-threatening. Enabling mothers to cope, they clearly promote family welfare but only by undermining individual health. They thus reflect, in a particularly sharp way, the conflicts that go with caring for health in circumstances of hardship.

Notes

1. African–Caribbean women quoted in Eyles and Donovan (1990), pp.65–6.

2. Mother quoted in Graham (1980), p.45.
3. Mother quoted in Popay (1992), p.114.
4. Mother quoted in Eyles and Donovan (1990), pp.49–50.
5. Lone mother quoted in Daly (1988), pp.75–6.
6. Mother quoted in Cohen *et al.* (1992), p.70.
7. Lone mother quoted in Cohen *et al.* (1992), p.88.
8. Lone mother, unpublished data from Graham (1985).
9. Lone mother and married mother quoted in Miller (1990), pp.39 and 83.
10. Mother quoted in Cohen *et al.* (1992), p.71.
11. Lone mothers, Graham, unpublished data.
12. Ibid.
13. African–Caribbean and Asian women quoted in Eyles and Donovan (1990), p.81.
14. Woman quoted in Gabe and Thorogood (1986), p.746.
15. Lone mother quoted in Graham (1988a), p.379.
16. Lone mother quoted in J. Wells (1987), p.12.
17. Lone mother, Graham, unpublished data.
18. Mother on income support, Graham, unpublished data.
19. Cohabiting mother quoted in Graham (1988a), p.379.
20. Graham, unpublished data.
21. Mothers quoted in Simms and Smith (1986), pp.78–9.
22. Two mothers quoted in Graham (1988b), p.7.

CHAPTER 10

CHILDREN'S HEALTH

10.1 Introduction

Earlier chapters have described how hardship frames and constrains what mothers can do for their children. Immigration laws make reunion increasingly hard for Asian families to achieve. Current housing policies are denying many mothers access to the homes they need for themselves and their children. The evidence reviewed in earlier chapters points to the way in which low income affects not only the quality of the home but living standards within it. For mothers struggling to make ends meet, the drive to economise means cutting back on items that they know are important for health. These health-promoting resources include not only food, but other material resources like fuel and transport, clothes and toys. Poverty does more than restrict access to material resources. It also restricts access to the events and experiences which make up the everyday lives of most children in Britain. School trips and family outings, bus journeys and meals out are sacrificed as mothers struggle both to protect basic necessities and service household debts.

Mothers have highlighted other health-costs of hardship. In the last chapter, their accounts recorded how caring on less than you need drains the energy of mothers. It leaves them searching for ways of keeping themselves as well as their families going, ways which – ironically – are often health damaging.

Living their lives within the timetable of other people's needs, women with children have provided a detailed catalogue of the toll that hardship takes on health. However, it is not women's accounts that stand as the official record of how and how much hardship hurts. It is official statistics and survey data which provide this record. These sources describe the absence rather than the presence of health: they give information on mortality, morbidity and use of welfare services (see Chapter 1). Of the various measures generated through the data-gathering processes of the state, it is those relating to deaths among children that are regarded as particularly sensitive indicators of the wealth and health of the population.

Before concluding the book's review of hardship and health in women's lives, this chapter briefly considers some of the official data on deaths among children. It begins by summarising the measures used before mapping out what they reveal about childhood deaths in Britain.

10.2 Measuring children's health

Those concerned with how standards of living and standards of health are linked have looked to official statistics on children's health. In particular, they have looked to statistics on deaths in infancy (Rodrigues and Botting, 1989). Deaths among children aged less than one year are included in the infant mortality statistics, while deaths among children aged over 1 and under 15 are recorded in statistics on childhood mortality.

Statistics on infant mortality are often further subdivided into neonatal mortality, which refers to deaths in the first 28 days of life, and post-neonatal mortality, which includes deaths in the remainder of the first year of life. Stillbirths, which are defined as foetal deaths after 28 weeks of gestation, are not included in the statistics on infant mortality (nor in neonatal mortality statistics). They are, however, included in perinatal mortality, a measure which covers stillbirths and deaths in the first week of life. These different categories of mortality are summarised in Table 10.1 on page 187.

In the search for measures of disadvantage, researchers have been restricted to the information recorded on birth and death certificates (see Chapter 1). This information includes details of the mother's marital status, age and area of residence at the time of her baby's birth. It also includes information on her country of birth. This provides an increasingly unreliable indicator of the ethnic identity of children because the vast majority of White,

Table 10.1 Statistics on mortality in childhood.

Category	Definition	Measure
Childhood mortality	Deaths at all ages over 1 year and under 15 years	Rate per 100,000 population
Infant mortality	Deaths at all ages under 1 year	Rate per 1000 live births
Post-neonatal mortality	Deaths at ages over 28 days and under 1 year	Rate per 1000 births
Neonatal mortality	Deaths in the first 28 days of life	Rate per 1000 live births
Perinatal mortality	Stillbirths and deaths in the first week of life	Rate per 1000 live and stillbirths
Stillbirths	Foetal deaths after 28 weeks of gestation	Rates per 1000 live and stillbirths

African–Caribbean and Asian children are born in Britain. None the less, it still provides a reasonably good proxy measure of the ethnic background of women of childbearing age. As noted in Chapter 2, while most White women over the age of 25 were born in the United Kingdom, the majority of African–Caribbean and Asian women in this age group are non-UK born.

It is social class that provides the most widely used measure of relative material advantage and disadvantage among Black and White children. As noted in Chapter 2, social class is measured through the Registrar General's classification of occupation, with children allocated a social class on the basis of their father's occupation. Most class analyses of infant mortality include only children born to married couples. None the less, the Registrar General's classification provides powerful evidence that poor material conditions cut deeply into the lives of children in Britain.

10.3 Patterns of infant mortality

Death rates are generally at their highest immediately after birth. They fall sharply throughout the first year of life and then continue to fall, though more slowly, through childhood. Death rates are at their lowest around the age of 8 for girls and 9 for boys, after which they rise gradually with age (Office of

Population Censuses and Surveys, 1991e). Across the age range, boys face a higher risk of death than girls. For example, among children aged 1 to 4, girls have a death rate of 36 per 100,000. The rate among boys is 44 per 100,000.

While sex differences are pronounced, class differences are sharper still. It is mothers in the poorest socioeconomic circumstances who are most likely to experience the death of a child in the first year of life. The class gradient in deaths among young children comes across powerfully in the data on infant mortality, summarised in Figure 10.1. It includes only children born within marriage, with their social class position ascribed on the basis of their father's occupation at the time the death was registered. Babies born into social class V have an infant mortality rate which, at 10.5 per 1000 live births, is nearly twice as high as that found among babies born into social class I, which has an infant mortality rate of 5.9 per 1000 (Office of Population Censuses and Surveys, 1992).

Looking within the period covered by infant mortality

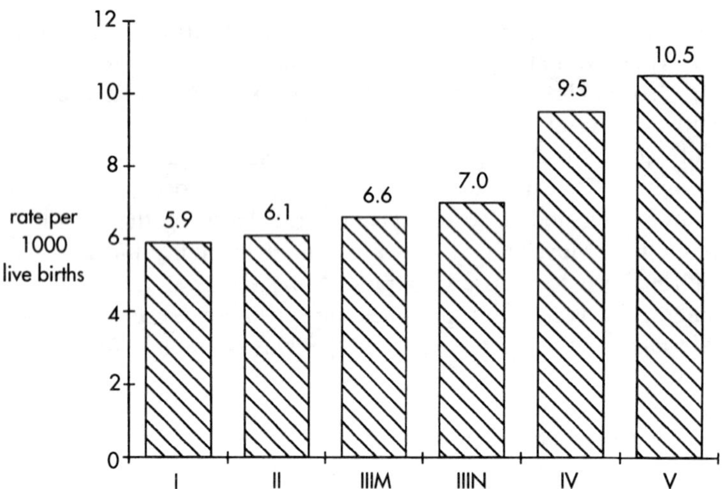

Figure 10.1 Infant mortality by father's social class (births within marriage only), England and Wales, 1989.

Source: Office of Population Censuses and Surveys (1992), derived from Table 5.

statistics, a similarly sharp class gradient emerges. Stillbirth rates are twice as high among babies born within marriage to fathers in social class V as among those born to fathers in social class I (Office of Population Censuses and Surveys, 1992). In the neonatal period, where deaths are seen as closely linked to the quality of medical care, class differences are less pronounced. However, the class gradient steepens in the post-neonatal period, a time when social and economic circumstances are seen to play a major role in child mortality (Rodrigues and Botting, 1989). Table 10.2 maps out the scale of class inequalities in stillbirth rates and in mortality among children under a year old.

The impact of social and material disadvantage comes across in other measures of social position. It is apparent in the patterns of infant mortality among babies born to single and married women, with single mothers significantly more likely to face the death of their baby in the first twelve months of life (Office of Population Censuses and Surveys, 1992). In the late 1980s, the infant mortality rate for babies born to married women was 7.7 per 1000 live births. Among non-married women registering the birth of their baby jointly with a partner, the rate was over a third higher at 10.5 per 1000. Single women who registered their baby's birth alone faced an infant mortality rate of 13.8, a rate 80 per cent higher than that found among babies born within marriage (Figure 10.2). As noted in Chapter 2, social class is meshed into marital status. Births to married couples are more common in social classes I and II, while births to single women, either living

Table 10.2 Stillbirths and infant deaths by father's social class (births within marriage only), England and Wales, 1989.

Social class	Stillbirths[a]	Perinatal deaths[a]	Neonatal deaths[b]	Postneonatal deaths[b]
I	3.0	5.8	3.9	2.0
II	3.8	6.9	4.0	2.1
IIIN	4.2	7.4	4.0	2.6
IIIM	4.4	7.7	4.4	2.6
IV	4.9	8.8	5.0	4.5
V	6.2	10.2	5.2	5.3

Note: Social class as defined by father's occupation at death registration.
[a] Rate per 1000 total births
[b] Rate per 1000 live births
Source: Office of Population Censuses and Surveys (1992), derived from Tables 1–4.

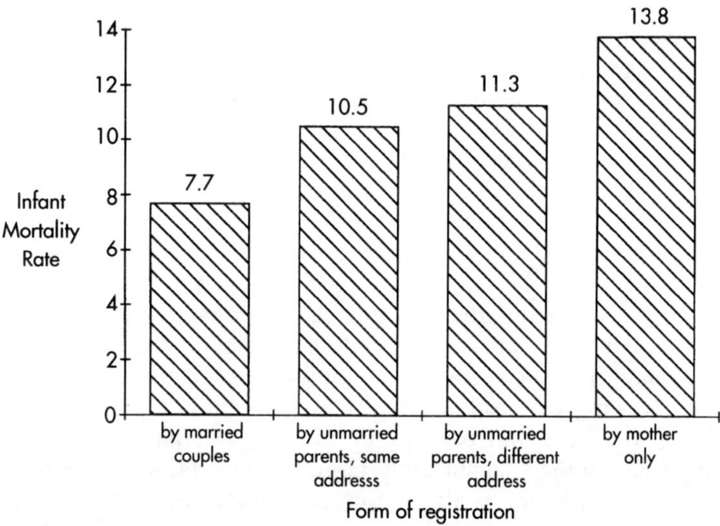

Figure 10.2 Infant mortality and marital status, England and Wales, 1987–9.

Source: Office of Population Censuses and Surveys (1992), p.xv.

on their own or with men, are more common among those whose occupation places them in social classes IV and V (Simms and Smith, 1986; Office of Population Censuses and Surveys, 1991c).

Social and economic disadvantage is also woven into the patterns of infant mortality among minority and majority ethnic groups. Taking mother's country of birth as a proxy measure of ethnic identity, Figure 10.3 maps out the patterns of infant deaths among women born within and outside the United Kingdom. While there are important exceptions, the dominant pattern is one in which babies born to mothers whose birthplace was the Indian subcontinent, Africa and the Caribbean, are less likely to survive the first year of life than babies of mothers born in the United Kingdom (Office of Population Censuses and Surveys, 1992). The low rates of infant mortality among Bangladeshi children represent one of these important exceptions. While born into one of the poorest communities in Britain, Bangladeshi children are less likely to die in the first year of life than other children. While Bangladeshi mothers probably know why their care protects their children against disadvantage, the reasons are

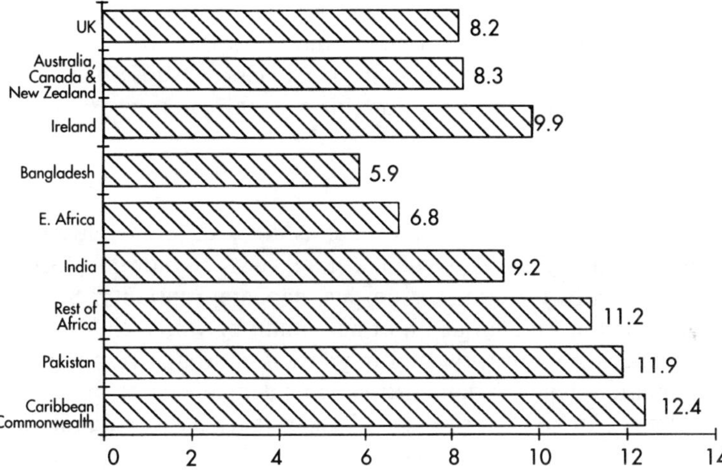

Figure 10.3 Infant mortality and mother's country of birth, England and Wales, 1989.

Source: Office of Population Censuses and Surveys (1992), derived from Table 12a.

little understood as yet by those who chart the patterns of child health in Britain.

These patterns, summarised in Figures 10.1 to 10.3 and Table 10.2, suggest that social disadvantage and deaths in infancy are closely related. Official data on the causes of deaths in infancy underline these links. In the neonatal period (the first month of life), it is 'congenital anomalies' and 'prematurity' which are recorded as the major causes of death. These two diagnostic categories account for 60 per cent of all neonatal deaths (Office of Population Censuses and Surveys, 1991e). Low birthweight plays an important part in these deaths. While only 6 in every 100 babies born to married couples have birthweights of less than 2500 grams, they make up nearly 60 per cent of the babies born within marriage who die in the first month of life (Office of Population Censuses and Surveys, 1992). It is mothers living in materially disadvantaged circumstances who are most at risk of having a baby whose weight falls below the 2500 gram threshold. Thus, single mothers are more at risk than married mothers and mothers whose birthplace was the Indian subcontinent are more at risk than mothers born in the United Kingdom. The links between disadvantage and birthweight are also captured in the class patterns of low birthweight among babies born to married women. It is married mothers in social class V whose babies are most likely to fall into the low birthweight category (Office of Population Censuses and Surveys, 1992).

In the post-neonatal period – between the end of the first month and the end of the first year of life – the information recorded on death certificates points to a different cluster of causes of mortality. It is sudden infant death syndrome (SIDS) that dominates the statistics on post-neonatal mortality. SIDS is defined as the 'sudden death of any infant or young child, which is unexpected by history, and in which a thorough post-mortem examination fails to demonstrate an adequate cause of death' (Beckwith, 1970). Over the last decade, there has been a marked increase in the SIDS rate and a corresponding decrease in deaths attributed to respiratory conditions. These trends are interpreted as a change in certifying habits, with deaths previously classified as having respiratory causes increasingly classified as SIDS (Rodrigues and Botting, 1989). Today, SIDS accounts for nearly half (46 per cent) of post-neonatal deaths. The next major cause of death, congenital anomalies, make up 17 per cent of deaths in the post-neonatal period (Office of Population Censuses and Surveys, 1991e).

While the major causes of mortality in the post-neonatal period are different from those associated with the first month of life, they remain ones which are deprivation related. Social and material disadvantage has been identified among the cluster of factors associated with SIDS. As Figure 10.4 records, it is babies born to fathers in social classes IV and V, and to mothers who are single, who are most at risk of facing death from SIDS (Office of Population Censuses and Surveys, 1992).

10.4 Patterns of childhood mortality

The class gradient in mortality in the first year of life continues through childhood. The risks of death among children aged 1 to 15 are significantly higher among boys and girls born to fathers in social class V than among those in social class I (Figure 10.5). The risks to life are no longer the ones which threaten the

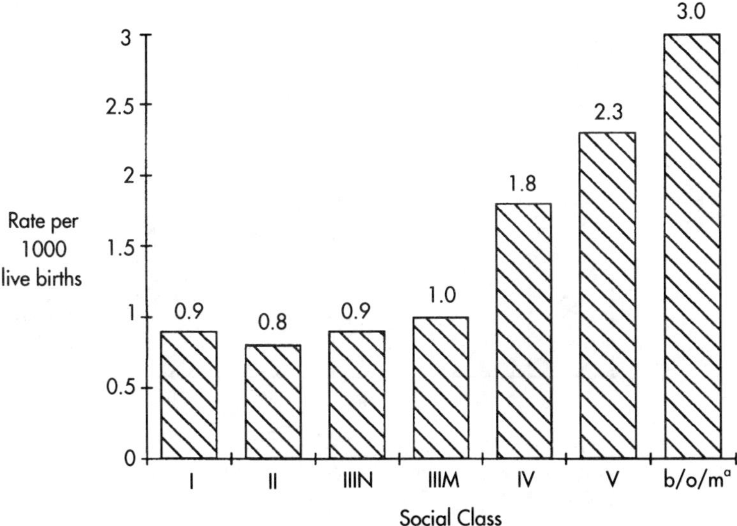

Figure 10.4 Post-neonatal deaths: sudden death, cause unknown, by father's social class and by births outside marriage, England and Wales, 1989.

[a] Births outside marriage.
Note: Data on fathers' social class includes births within marriage only.
Source: Office of Population Censuses and Surveys (1992), derived from Table 19.

survival of children under the age of 1. Among children over the age of 1, it is injuries and poisonings that are the largest single cause of death. They make up a progressively larger proportion of deaths as children get older. As Figure 10.6 indicates, injury and poisoning account for around one in four deaths among preschool children but over 40 per cent of deaths among children aged 10 to 14. By the time children reach this age group, injury and poisoning dwarfs the other main causes of death in childhood: cancer, nervous system diseases and congenital anomalies. Accidental deaths are more common among boys and are the main reason why death rates are higher in childhood among boys than girls (Office of Population Censuses and Surveys, 1988). Accidents (a category which includes violence)

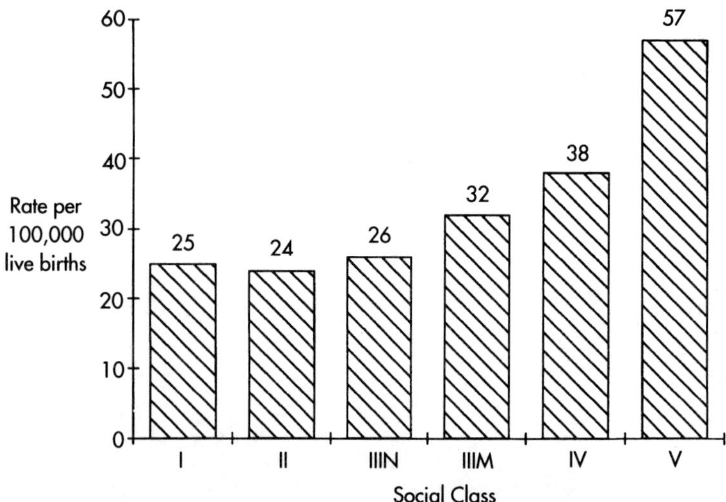

Figure 10.5 Mortality among boys aged 1 to 15 by father's social class, England and Wales, 1979–80 and 1982–3.

Source: Office of Population Censuses and Surveys (1988), derived from Table 2.6.

accounts for one quarter (24 per cent) of deaths among girls aged 1 to 14, but over a third (34 per cent) of deaths among boys in this age group (Dunnell, 1990).

It is accidental deaths that display the steepest class gradient in childhood. The death rates for all causes of childhood mortality is about twice as high among children born into social class V as it is among children born into social class I; when accidental deaths are singled out, mortality rates are three times as high among children in social class V (Office of Population Censuses and Surveys, 1988). The differences are particularly marked among pedestrian deaths and deaths in fires.

However, death is only part of the toll of accidents. Long term and permanent disability is more common than death (Quick, 1991). While the official data-collecting agencies do not monitor the long term effects of accidents on children's health, it has been estimated that over 2000 children a year are permanently disabled following accidents.

Childhood deaths and injuries from accidents have often been explained in terms of the characteristics of the children to whom

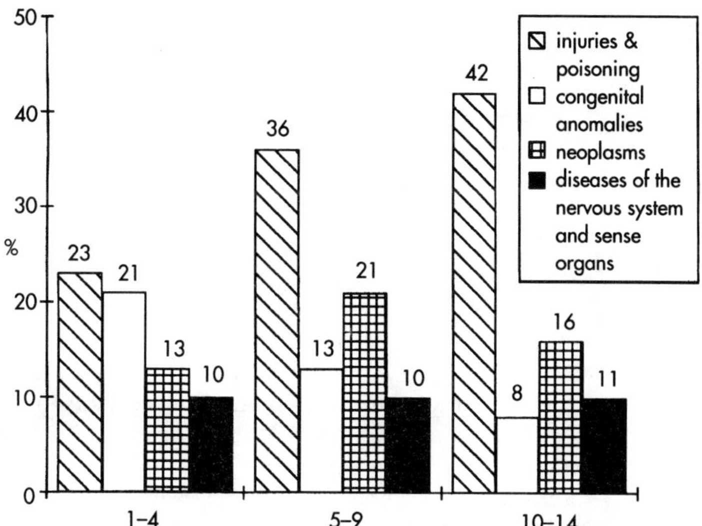

Figure 10.6 Selected causes of death among children aged 1 to 14, England and Wales, 1989.

Source: Office of Population Censuses and Surveys (1991e), derived from Figure D.

they happen and the parents who fail to prevent them. The underlying concept was one of 'accident proneness', a concept that conveys the idea that some children invite danger – and some parents neglect their safety. While such perspectives are still influential, there is now a sizable body of research which challenges this victim-blaming approach (Constantinides, 1988). This research has drawn attention to the dangers that lurk, not in the attitudes and behaviour of children and their parents, but in the environments in which families live. As one researcher put it, 'there are effective ways to keep our children healthy and whole . . . exhorting parents to be careful is not one of them' (Baker, 1981).

Among preschool children, it is the home that is the most likely setting for accidents. Earlier chapters have described the poor material conditions experienced by many families and how these conditions are associated with symptoms of physical and emotional ill-health among children. Accidents are part of a web of health hazards facing children growing up in poor and poorly designed housing. As the accounts included in Chapter 3 indicate, homes have built-in hazards which mothers need to shield their children against. Preventive measures, however, often have a hefty price-tag attached. For example, a fireguard costing £22 represents nearly a third of the weekly income support received by a lone mother over 18 with one child under 11. A stair-gate, which currently retails at around £25, would consume half the week's income support of a lone mother under 18 bringing up her baby on the lower rate of benefit (see Table 7.1).

Mothers' perceptions of risk and their fears for the safety of their children are reflected in hospital statistics on admissions to accident and emergency departments. About half a million children under the age of 5 attend accident and emergency departments each year for injuries resulting from accidents in the home (Alwash and McCarthy, 1988). A study based on a West London hospital illustrates how home environments are linked to the risk of accidents. Accidents to children were significantly more common in families in rented accommodation, in families in shared accommodation and in families in accommodation where there were more than 1.5 people per room. These features, in turn, were closely related to social class, with four times as many children in social class V as in social class I admitted to accident departments. The study found no difference among the different ethnic groups represented in the study, which included both Asian and African–Caribbean families. As the authors concluded, 'social disadvantage seems to be more important than ethnicity as a determinant of accidents to children in the home' (Alwash and McCarthy, 1988, p.1450).

Other studies have highlighted how social disadvantage is reflected in the risks of injury faced by young children. One recent study carried out in Haringey, in north London, focused on accidents to children under 5 for which medical attention was sought. The vast majority of the children (72 per cent) sustained their injury at home. The remaining injuries typically occurred on the streets (9 per cent) or on waste or recreation grounds (8 per cent). Accidents were much more common among children living in areas in the borough where disadvantage was clustered. There was a fourfold difference in the accident rate among children in the affluent and disadvantaged parts of the borough. The higher accident rate in the eastern half of Haringey was associated with a range of poverty indicators, including living in overcrowded accommodation and in property owned by the council or housing association. Being part of a family classified within social classes IV and V, and with a head of household who was unemployed, was also significantly related to the risk of accidental injury (Constantinides, 1988).

Social disadvantage is the thread that also runs through the patterns of mortality among older children. Among children over 5, it is motor vehicles that are the major cause of accidental death, accounting for over half of all deaths from accidents (Quick, 1991). Most of these traffic-related deaths occur to children hit by vehicles, either as pedestrians or cyclists, rather than to children travelling in them. Over 40 per cent of all fatal accidents to children under the age of 15 are pedestrian and pedal-cyclist deaths.

These pedestrian and pedal-cyclist deaths are concentrated among older children, in the 10 to 14 age range. Children of this age are typically independent road users who are not as closely supervised by parents as younger children. Reflecting the particular risks faced by older children, the evidence suggests that, while traffic accidents caused fewer deaths among children under 10, road deaths among those in the 10 to 14 age group have been increasing (Quick, 1991). Like accidental deaths more generally, there is a sharp class gradient in childhood deaths from traffic accidents. Families headed by an unskilled manual head of household are least likely to own a car (Office of Population Censuses and Surveys, 1991a). Yet, ironically the children in these households are the ones most often killed on the road (Office of Population Censuses and Surveys, 1988). As Bob Holman notes, 'children whose parents can not afford a car are knocked over by those who can' (Holman, 1991, p.7).

The statistics on accidental deaths in childhood, reflect, in sharp and stark ways, the health risks that go with material disadvantage in Britain. Like the other measures of children's health reviewed in this chapter, they provide a postscript to the aspects of women's lives explored in the main part of the book. It is a postscript that underlines the messages that women have conveyed about motherhood. It confirms the fact that hardship and health are intimately connected in the family lives of mothers and their children.

CHAPTER 11

CONCLUDING COMMENTS

This book has focused on the domestic lives of women with children. It has mapped out the common domestic responsibilities that mothers carry and the different domestic circumstances in which they carry them.

In describing the responsibilities and circumstances of mothers' lives, the chapters have tried to stay close to the understandings that women have of what they do and how they live. However, the book has worked with data constructed in ways which can obscure what women want to say about themselves. What passes as scientific knowledge in Britain has been built up through a set of data-collection methods where minority voices can go unheard. It has been constructed, too, through measures of social position which represent diversity and inequality in restricted ways. Measures of social class, 'race' and sexuality, like those that tap the experience of being disabled and non-disabled, can mask what women are most concerned about. They can simultaneously leave out what is most valued and what is most oppressive about being working class and Black, lesbian and disabled. Mainstream research can be poorly tuned into how women experience and organise their domestic lives.

Although mainstream research can miss and misrepresent what goes on in women's lives, it provides the major part of what is known about motherhood. It is official statistics and social surveys which record mothers' housing circumstances and employment patterns, the composition of their households and how much money comes into them. It is these data sources, too, which track the distribution of ill-health among mothers and the patterns of death among their children. Further, the evidence derived from statistics and surveys carries an authority which is rarely accorded to the accounts that women give of their lives.

The book has therefore worked with the recognised sources of information. It has tried to piece together an account of what women do in and for their families by grounding official and survey data in what women have said about their lives. The result is a patchwork, frayed at the edges in places and with a few pieces missing. But it is a patchwork which is complete enough for the patterns within it to be clear.

The patterns underline how caring for families is a deeply gendered experience. It is something many women but few men do. In households with young children, the sexual division of domestic labour is at its sharpest. In these households, it is women who take responsibility for the children and for the domestic routines that promote their health and development. It is a responsibility which most women anticipate and welcome: taking care of their children is what being a mother means. However, taking care of children in hardship is increasingly what being a mother is about.

> I have actually had to swallow my pride till it hurts. . . . It makes me feel like a complete failure because I had such high ideals. . . . I wanted to give my children the best, not to the point of spoiling them, but just so they could, you know, have confidence in themselves. So when I can't do that it makes me feel I'm failing.[1]

The official and unofficial sources of information used in this book have recorded the increasing scale of material hardship in mothers' lives. The trends in homelessness among families are upward. More mothers are bringing up children in low-income households and on benefit. More are caring in the face of credit commitments they cannot meet and debts they cannot repay. Motherhood is structured around an unending conflict between caring enough and economising enough, trying to be a good enough mother who simultaneously meets and denies her children's needs.

> It's a very depressing thought to think we might have to spend maybe the next five years on social security. . . . It's a very disheartening, depressing thought to bring your new baby into the world, because when I had him, do you know one of my first thoughts was, 'Isn't he beautiful . . . oh I'm so happy, oh God,

> how am I going to manage to bring him up and keep him fed and clothed decently'. That sums it up for me.[2]

The records that mothers have kept of their lives describe how material hardship enters the household through the routines that they develop to care for their family's health. It makes its way into families through the food women buy and the clothes they borrow, through the outings they do not take their children on and the school trips they cannot afford. Hardship enters family life by limiting it to one warm room and by restricting where parents and children sleep, and whether they can sleep in a bed of their own.

> I'm very afraid these days; I get Gregory (son) to fetch the post for me. I hate those brown envelopes that come every month for gas, rates etc. . . . The whole house is furnished from car boot and jumble sales, handouts and bits that were left by the previous owners. I can't afford to heat more than one room at a time, and still have bare floorboards in my bedroom. Gregory, the cat and I all sleep in the same bed with two quilts, socks, T-shirts and a hot water bottle . . .[3]

It is not only material hardship which tracks its way through mothers' lives. Mothers confront, and try to contain, other kinds of inequality as they care for their children. Class inequalities leave working class mothers searching for ways of protecting children from accidental injury in cramped and poorly designed homes, and from accidental death on the roads. Many lone mothers find they have to build new lives for themselves in circumstances not of their choosing. Mothers in one- and two-parent families who are Black and disabled, too, are engaged in a process of building lives that resist inequality. Like lesbian mothers, their caring routines provide a space in which children can grow up strong. Struggling with and for children is not always a negative experience. It often has a creative side, a sense of 'embarking on an adventure together of how to try and do things differently' (Ross, 1988, p.182).

> Being a Black woman I had had good preparation for the possibility of a struggle because people in a powerless position always have to know the ins and outs and the to-ings and fro-ings of the people with power: you have to, if you're going to survive. I

> was strong and part of my strength was support from the kids themselves and my friends . . .[4]

The way women care not only protects others; it helps them cope too. It releases resources for mothers to care for themselves, to keep going when life feels like it is dishing out more than they can take. Family, friends and partners can provide some mothers with what they need to survive. Cigarettes offer a more contradictory kind of support but one, none the less, that is an essential part of how many mothers get through each day.

> I've faced a whole series of things. The courts, solicitors, DHSS. I just went down to the doctors then and I was on pills for nerves, then after a year, I started to get things together and it was a lot better. It was just – either you go down, and you end up having a nervous breakdown and your children are taken away from you, or you end up that you start to cope more. You get things back more on an even keel. Be more sort of so you depend on other people. You can't always cope on your own. And when you start doing that, making friends and being involved, I thought it was a lot better for all of us, my kids and myself. And things started to go from worse to better.[5]

The patchwork stitched out of the official and unofficial data on women's lives suggests that containing hardship and resisting inequality takes a heavy toll on the health of parents and children. But, despite the toll, women do not give in. The accounts recorded in this book underline how many mothers make it through each day and bring their families with them.

> I'm not saying it was easy to start with, the kids were in a state and so was I. But despite all the difficulties the kids became more settled and I felt immensely grateful that they trusted me and relied on me to cope. Then came a time when I realised that not only was I coping on my own, I was actually enjoying it. No rows about who does what. I had to do it all, so I did it and I felt stronger and better about myself as a result. I don't want to be a martyr or get off on being a superwoman. I'll accept any offers of help any friends care to make now but I think it was important to prove to myself that I could cope on my own and feel strengthened, not weakened, by doing so.[6]

While the fabric of their lives often wears thin, it is resilient enough to hold them, their children, their partners and their friends together. Mothers emerge from the patchwork of their lives as survivors. They are not the powerless victims of poverty and oppression but are agents of their lives, actively engaged in caring for health and struggling against hardship.

> Even before she was born, it's always been stressful, 'cos my dad left me, me brother's in prison, I married her dad, got beaten up, left him and, believe it or not, since I've got older – and I know it sounds stupid 'cos I am starting to look grey – but it's gotten better. But now, oh I don't know, now I've had her – she's what I've always wanted – things are getting better. They've got to get better from what they were.[7]

Notes

1. Mother on benefit quoted in Cohen *et al.* (1992), p.72.
2. Ibid., p.69.
3. Taking Liberties Collective (1989), pp.29–30.
4. Ross (1988), p.176.
5. Lone mother, unpublished data from Graham (1985).
6. Taking Liberties Collective (1989), p.32.
7. Lone mother, Graham, unpublished data.

REFERENCES

Abberley, P. (1990) *Handicapped by Numbers: A critique of the OPCS disability surveys* (Bristol: Occasional Papers in Sociology No.9, Bristol Polytechnic)

Afshar, H. (1989) 'Gender roles and the "moral economy of kin" among Pakistani women in West Yorkshire', *New Community*, vol.15, no.2, pp.211–25

Allen, S. and Wolkowitz, C. (1987) *Homeworking: Myths and realities* (London: Macmillan)

Alwash, R. and McCarthy, M. (1988) 'Accidents in the home among children under 5: ethnic differences or social disadvantage?', *British Medical Journal*, vol.296, pp.1450–3

Baker, S. (1981) 'Childhood injuries: the community approach to prevention', *Journal of Public Health Policy*, vol.2, no.3, pp.235–46

Baldwin, S. (1985) *The Costs of Caring: Families with disabled children* (London: Routledge & Kegan Paul)

Barr, N. and Coulter, F. (1990) 'Social security: solution or problem?', in Hills, J. (ed.) *The State of Welfare: The welfare state in Britain since 1974* (Oxford: Clarendon Press)

Barry, J. (1991) *Child Care at Work*, MSc dissertation, University of Bristol: Faculty of Social Science

Bebbington, A.C. (1991) 'The expectations of life without disability in England and Wales: 1976–88', *Population Trends*, vol.66, pp.26–9

Beckett, H. (1986) 'Adolescent identity development', in Wilkinson, S. (ed.) *Feminist Social Psychology* (Milton Keynes: Open University Press)

Beckwith, J.B. (1970) 'Definition of sudden infant death syndrome', in Bergman, A.B., Beckwith, J.B., and Ray, C.G. (eds) *Sudden Infant Death Syndrome* (Seattle: University of Washington)

Bennett, F. (1992) 'Childcare costs', *Benefits*, no.5, pp.41–2.

Berthoud, R. (1989) *Credit, Debt and Poverty* (London: Social Security Advisory Committee, Research Paper 1, HMSO)

Berthoud, R. and Kempson, E. (1992) *Credit and Debt: The PSI report* (London: Policy Studies Institute)

Beuret, K. (1991) 'Women and transport', in Maclean, M. and Groves, D. (eds) *Women's Issues in Social Policy* (London: Routledge)

Bhabha, J., Klug, F. and Shutter, S. (eds) (1985) *Worlds Apart: Women under immigration and nationality law*, The Women, Immigration and Nationality Group, (London: Pluto Press)

Bhachu, P. (1988) 'Apni marzi kardhi. Home and work: Sikh women in Britain', in Westwood, S. and Bhachu, P. (eds) *Enterprising Women: Ethnicity, economy and gender relations* (London: Routledge)

Bhachu, P. (1991) 'Culture, ethnicity and class among Punjabi Sikh women in 1990s Britain', *New Community*, vol.17, no.3, pp.401–12

Binney, V., Harkell, G. and Nixon, J. (1985) 'Refuges and housing for battered women', in Pahl, J. (ed.) *Private Violence and Public Policy* (London: Routledge & Kegan Paul)

Blackburn, C. (1991) *Poverty and Health: Working with families* (Milton Keynes: Open University Press)

Blaxter, M. (1990) *Health and Lifestyles* (London: Routledge)

Bolchever, S., Stewart, S. and Clyde, G. (1990) 'Consumer credit: investigating the loan sharks', *Trading Standards Review*, vol.98, no.1, pp.18–22

Bone, M. and Meltzer, H. (1989) *The Prevalence of Disability Among Children* (London: OPCS Surveys of Disability in Great Britain, Report 3, HMSO)

Bonnerjea, L. and Lawton, J. (1987) *Homelessness in Brent* (London: Policy Studies Institute)

Booth, H. (1988) 'Identifying ethnic origin: the past, present and future of official data production', in Bhat, A., Carr-Hill, R. and Ohri, S. (eds) *Britain's Black Population* (Aldershot, Hants: Gower)

Boulton, M.G. (1983) *On Being A Mother: A study of women with pre-school children* (London: Tavistock)

Bradshaw, J. (1990) *Child Poverty and Deprivation in the UK* (London: National Children's Bureau)

Bradshaw, J. and Holmes, H. (1989) *Living on the Edge: A study of the living standards of families on benefit in Tyne and Wear* (London: Child Poverty Action Group)

Bradshaw, J. and Millar, J. (1991) *Lone Parent Families in the UK* (London: DSS Research Report No. 6, HMSO)

Bradshaw, J. and Morgan, J. (1987) *Budgeting on Benefit: The consumption of families on social security* (London: Family Policy Studies Centre)

Brah, A. (1992) 'Women of South Asian origin in Britain: issues and concerns', in Braham, P., Rattansi, A. and Skellington, R. (eds) *Racism and Anti-racism: Inequalities, opportunities and policies* (London: Sage Publications)

Brannen, J. and Moss, P. (1988) *New Mothers at Work: Employment and childcare*, (London: Unwin Hyman)

Brown, C. (1984) *Black and White Britain: The third PSI survey* (Aldershot, Hants: Gower)

Brown, C. (1990) 'Race relations and discrimination', *Policy Studies*, vol.11, no.2: pp.47–52

Brown, G. and Harris, T. (1978) *The Social Origins of Depression* (London: Tavistock)

Brown, J. (1988) *Child Benefit: Investing in the future* (London: Child Poverty Action Group)

Browne, S., Connors, D. and Stern, N. (eds) (1985) *With the Power of Each Breath – A disabled woman's anthology* (San Francisco: Cleis Press)

Bryan, B., Dadzie, S. and Scafe, S. (1985) *The Heart of the Race: Black women's lives in Britain* (London: Virago)

Carr-Hill, R. and Drew, D. (1988) 'Blacks, police and crime' in Bhat, A., Carr-Hill, R. and Ohri, S. (eds) *Britain's Black Population* (Aldershot, Hants: Gower)

Central Statistical Office (1988) *Social Trends 18* (London: HMSO)

Central Statistical Office (1991) *Family Spending: A report on the 1990 Family Expenditure Survey* (London: HMSO)

Central Statistical Office (1992) *Social Trends 22* (London: HMSO)

Chandler, J. (1991) *Women Without Husbands: An exploration of the margins of marriage* (London: Macmillan)

Charles, N. and Kerr, M. (1988) *Women, Food and Families* (Manchester: Manchester University Press)

Child Poverty Action Group (1992) *National Welfare Benefits Handbook 1992/3* (London: Child Poverty Action Group)

City of Liverpool (1991) *The Liverpool Quality of Life Survey* (Liverpool: Liverpool City Council)

Clark E. (1989) *Young Single Mothers Today* (London: National Council for One Parent Families)

Cohen, R. (1988) 'Single payments surveyed', in Cohen, R. and Tarpey, M. (eds) *Single Payments: The disappearing safety net* (London: Child Poverty Action Group)

Cohen, R. (1991a) *Just About Surviving. Life on Income Support: Debt and the social fund* (London: Family Service Units)

Cohen, R. (1991b) '"If you have everything second-hand, you feel second-hand": bringing up children on income support', *FSU Quarterly*, vol.46, pp.25–41

Cohen, R. (1991c) *Just About Surviving. Life on Income Support: Quality of life and the impact of local services* (London: Family Service Units)

Cohen, R., Coxall, J., Craig, G. and Sadiq-Sangster, A. (1992) *Hardship Britain: Being poor in the 1990s* (London: Child Poverty Action Group)

Cohen, S. (1985) 'Anti-semitism, immigration controls and the welfare state', *Critical Social Policy*, vol.13, pp.73–92

Coles, A. (1990) 'Mortgage possessions and money advice – building society views', *Housing Review*, vol.39, no.14, pp.88–90

Constantinides, P. (1988) 'Safe at home? Children's accidents and inequalty', *Radical Community Medicine*, Spring, pp.31–4

Conway, J. (1988) *Prescription for Poor Health: The crisis for homeless families* (London: London Food Commission, Maternity Alliance, SHAC, Shelter)

Cooper, J. (1991) 'Births outside marriage: recent trends and associated demographic and social changes', *Population Trends*, vol.63, pp.8–18

Cornwell, J. (1984) *Hard-earned Lives: Accounts of health and illness from East London* (London: Tavistock)

Cox, B.D. (ed.) (1987) *The Health and Lifestyle Survey* (London: Health Promotion Research Trust)

Craig, G. (1991) 'Life on the Social', *Social Work Today*, vol.22, pp.16–17

Craig, G. and Glendinning, C. (1990) *Missing the Target* (Ilford, Essex: Barnados)

Craig, P. (1991) 'Costs and benefits: a review of research on take-up of income-related benefits', *Journal of Social Policy*, vol.20, no.4, pp.537–65

Croghlan, R. (1991) 'First-time mothers' accounts of inequality in the division of labour', *Feminism and Psychology*, vol.1, no.2, pp.221–46

Crow, G. and Hardey, M. (1991) 'The housing strategies of lone parents', in Crow, G. and Hardey, M. (eds) *Lone Parenthood* (London: Harvester Wheatsheaf)

Cullen, I. (1979) 'Urban social policy and the problems of family life: the use of an extended diary method to inform decision analysis', in Harris, C. (ed.) *The Sociology of the Family: New directions for Britain* (Keele, Staffs: Sociological Review Monograph 28, University of Keele)

Currer, C. (1991) 'Understanding the mothers' viewpoint: the case of Pathan women in Britain', in Wyke, S. and Hewison, J. (eds) *Child Health Matters* (Milton Keynes: Open University Press)

Daly, M. (1988) *Money Lending and Low Income Families* (Dublin: Combat Poverty Agency)

Daly, M. (1989) *Women and Poverty* (Dublin: Attic Press)

Department of Health (1989) *On the State of the Public Health for the Year 1988* (London: HMSO)

Department of Health and Social Security (1985) *Reform of Social Security*, vol.2, Cmnd 9518 (London: HMSO)

Department of Social Security (1992a) *Social Security Statistics 1991* (London: HMSO)

Department of Social Security (1992b) *Households Below Average Income: A statistical analysis 1979–1988/9* (London: HMSO)

Devis, T. (1990) 'The expectation of life in England and Wales', *Population Trends*, vol.60, pp.23–4

Dex, S. (1984) *Women's Work Histories: An analysis of the women and employment survey* (London: Research Paper No. 46, Department of Employment)

Diamond, I. and Clarke, S. (1989) 'Demographic patterns among Britain's ethnic groups', in Joshi, H. (ed.) *The Changing Population of Britain* (Oxford: Blackwell)

Ditch, J., Pickles, S. and Whiteford, P. (1992) *The New Structure of Child Benefit* (London: Coalition for Child Benefit)

Dobash, R.E. and Dobash, R.P. (1980) *Violence Against Wives: A case against patriarchy* (Shepton Mallet: Open Books)

Doyal, L. (1990) 'Waged work and women's wellbeing', *Women's Studies International Forum*, vol.13, no.6, pp.587–604

Drury, B. (1991) 'Sikh girls and the maintenance of an ethnic culture', *New Community*, vol.17, no.3, pp.387–99

Duffy, K.B. and Lincoln, I.C. (1990) *Earnings and Ethnicity* (Leicester: Leicester City Council)

Dunnell, K. (1990) 'Monitoring children's health', *Population Trends*, vol.60, pp.16–22

Durward, L. (1990) *Traveller Mothers and Their Babies* (London: Maternity Alliance)

Eekelaar, J. and Maclean, M. (1985) *Maintenance After Divorce* (Oxford: Oxford University Press)

Ellis, J. (1992) 'To great applause', in Morris, J. (ed.) *Alone Together: Voices of Single Mothers* (London: Women's Press)

Employment Gazette (1990) 'Women in the labour market', *Employment Gazette*, vol.98, no.12, December, pp.619–43

Employment Gazette (1991) 'Ethnic origins and the labour market', *Employment Gazette*, vol.99, no.2, February, pp.59–72

Ermisch, J. (1989) 'Divorce: economic antecedents and aftermath', in Joshi, H. (ed.) *The Changing Population of Britain* (Oxford: Blackwell)

Evason, E. (1980) *Just Me and the Kids: A study of single parent families in Northern Ireland* (Belfast: Equal Opportunities Commission)

Evason, E. (1982) *Hidden Violence* (Belfast: Farset Press)

Eyles, J. and Donovan, J. (1990) *The Social Effects of Health Policy* (Aldershot: Avebury)

Family Policy Studies Centre (1990) *Family Finances* (London: Family Policy Studies Centre)

Feminist Arts News (1989) 'Disability arts: The real missing culture', *Feminist Arts News*, vol.2, no.10

Fenton, S. (1985) *Race, Health and Welfare* (Bristol: Department of Sociology, University of Bristol)

Ford, J. (1988) *The Indebted Society* (London: Routledge)

Ford, J. (1991) *Consuming Credit: Debt and poverty in the UK* (London: Child Poverty Action Group)

Fulop, N.S. (1992) *Gender, Parenthood and Health: A study of mothers' and fathers' experiences of health and illness*, PhD Thesis, Institute of Education, University of London

Gabe, J. and Thorogood, N. (1986) 'Prescribed drug use and the management of everyday life: the experiences of black and white working-class women', *Sociological Review*, vol.34, no.4, pp.737–72

Ginnety, P. (1985) *Moyard: A health profile* (Belfast : Moyard Health Group)

Ginsberg, N. (1992) 'Racism and housing: concepts and reality', in Braham, P., Rattansi, A. and Skellington, R. (eds) *Racism and Anti-racism: Inequalities, opportunities and policies* (London: Sage)

Glastonbury, M. (1979) 'The best kept secret – how working class women live and what they know', *Women's Studies International Quarterly*, vol.2, pp.171–81

Glendinning, C. (1983) *Unshared Care: Parents and their disabled children* (London: Routledge & Kegan Paul)

Goodman, B. (1980) 'Some mothers are lesbians' in Norman, E. and Muncuso, A. (eds) *Women's Issues and Social Work Practice* (Itasca, USA: Peacock Publishers)

Gordon, P. (1991) 'Forms of exclusion: citizenship, race and poverty' in Becker, S. (ed.) *Windows Of Opportunity: Public policy and the poor* (London: Child Poverty Action Group)

Gordon, P. and Newnham, A. (1985) *Passport to Benefits? Racism in social security* (London: Child Poverty Action Group)

Gordon, T. (1990) *Feminist Mothers* (London: Routledge)

Graham, H. (1980) 'Mothers' accounts of anger and aggression towards their babies', in Frude, N. (ed.) *Psychological Approaches to Child Abuse* (London: Batsford)

Graham, H. (1985) *Caring for the Family* (Milton Keynes: Faculty of Social Sciences, Open University)

Graham, H. (1986) *Caring for the Family*, (London: Research Report No. I, Health Education Council)

Graham, H. (1987a) 'Being poor: perceptions and coping strategies of lone mothers', in Brannen, J. and Wilson, G. (eds) *Give and Take in Families: Studies in resource distribution* (London: Allen & Unwin)

Graham, H. (1987b) 'Women's poverty and caring', in Glendinning, C. and Millar, J. (eds) *Women and Poverty in Britain* (Brighton: Wheatsheaf Books)

Graham, H. (1987c) 'Women's smoking and family health', *Social Science and Medicine*, vol.25, no.1, pp.47–56

Graham, H. (1988a) 'Women and smoking in the United Kingdom: implications for health promotion', *Health Promotion*, vol.3, no.4, pp.371–82

Graham, H. (1988b) 'Child health: mother's heartache', *Maternity Action*, vol.36, pp.6–7

Graham, H. (1992a) *Smoking Among Working Class Mothers With Children* (Coventry: Department of Applied Social Studies, University of Warwick)

Graham, H. (1992b) 'Budgeting for health: mothers in low-income households', in Glendinning, C. and Millar, J. (eds) *Women and Poverty in Britain, the 1990s* (London: Harvester Wheatsheaf)

Green, H. (1988) *Informal Carers* (London: HMSO)

Gregory, S. (1991) 'Challenging motherhood: mothers and their deaf children' in Phoenix, A., Woollett, A. and Lloyd, E. (eds) *Motherhood: Meanings, practices and ideologies* (London: Sage)

Greve, J. (1991) *Homelessness in Britain* (London: Rowntree Foundation)

Grewal, S., Kay, J., Landor, L., Lewis, G. and Parmar, P. (eds) (1988) *Charting the Journey: Writings by black and third world women* (London: Sheba Feminist Publishers)

Hakim, C. (1987) *Home-based Work in Britain* (London: Department of Employment Research Paper No. 60, HMSO)

Hall Carpenter Archives/Lesbian Oral History Group (1989) *Inventing Ourselves: Lesbian Life Stories* (London: Routledge)

Hall, S. (1991) 'Ethnicity: identity and difference', *Radical America*, vol.23, no.4, pp.9–13

Hanscombe, G.E. and Forster, J. (1981) *Rocking the Cradle: Lesbian mothers: A challenge in family living* (London: Peter Owen)

Hardey, M. and Glover, J. (1991) 'Income, employment, daycare and lone parenthood', in Hardey, M. and Crow, G. (eds) *Lone Parenthood* (London: Harvester Wheatsheaf)

Haskey, J. (1984) 'Social class and socio-economic differentials in divorce in England and Wales', *Population Studies*, vol.38, pp.419–38

Haskey, J. (1989a) 'Families and households of the ethnic minority and white populations of Great Britain', *Population Trends*, vol.57, pp.8–19

Haskey, J. (1989b) 'Current prospects for the proportion of marriages ending in divorce', *Population Trends*, vol.55, pp.34–7

Haskey, J. (1990) 'The ethnic minority populations of Great Britain: estimates by ethnic group and country of birth', *Population Trends*, vol.60, pp.35–8

Haskey, J. (1991a) 'Estimated numbers and demographic characteristics of one-parent families in Great Britain', *Population Trends*, vol.65, pp.35–47

Haskey, J. (1991b) 'Lone parenthood and demographic change', in Hardey, M. and Crow, G. (eds) *Lone Parenthood* (London: Harvester Wheatsheaf)

Heady, P. and Smyth, M. (1989) *Living Standards During Unemployment*, Vol.I (London: HMSO)

Henderson, J. and Karn, V. (1987) *Race, Class and State Housing: Inequality in the allocation of public housing in Britain* (Aldershot: Gower)

Hicks, C. (1988) *Who Cares: Looking after people at home* (London: Virago Press)

Hills, J. and Mullings, B. (1990) 'Housing: a decent home for all at a price within their means?', in Hills, J. (ed.) *The State of Welfare: The Welfare State in Britain since 1974* (Oxford: Clarendon Press)

Hobbs, S., Lavalette, M. and McKechnie, J. (1992) 'The emerging problem of child labour', *Critical Social Policy*, vol.34, pp.93–105

Holman, B. (1991) 'It's no accident', *Poverty*, vol.80, pp.6–8

Homer, M., Leonard, A.E. and Taylor, M.P. (1984) *Private Violence: Public shame* (Middlesborough: Cleveland Refuge and Aid for Women and Children)

Hope, S. (1992) 'Becoming a single person', in Morris, J. (ed.) *Alone Together: Voices of single mothers* (London: Women's Press)

House of Commons Home Affairs Committee (1986) *Bangladeshis in Britain*, Session 1986–7, vol.I (London: HMSO)

House of Commons (1991) *Low Income Statistics: Households below average income tables 1988* (London: HMSO)

Hughes, C. (1991) *Stepparents: Wicked or wonderful?* (Aldershot: Avebury)

Hunt, S.M. (1990) 'Emotional distress and bad housing', *Health and Hygiene*, vol.11, pp.72–9

Hunt, S.M., Martin, C.J., Platt, S., Lewis, C. and Morris, G. (1988) *Damp Housing, Mould Growth and Health Status* (Edinburgh: Research Unit in Health and Behavioural Change, University of Edinburgh)

Huws, V., Hurstfield, J. and Holtmatt, R. (1989) *What Price Flexibility*? (London: Low Pay Unit)

Jones, C. (1991) 'Birth statistics 1990' *Population Trends*, vol.65, pp.9–15

Joshi, H. (1989) 'The changing forms of women's economic dependency', in Joshi, H. (ed.) *The Changing Population of Britain* (Oxford: Blackwell)

Jowell, R., Witherspoon, S. and Brook, L. (1988) *British Social Attitudes*: *The 5th report* (Aldershot: Gower)

Jules, A. (1992) 'Feeling positive' in Morris, J. (ed.) *Alone Together*: *Voices of single mothers* (London: Women's Press)

Kemp, P. (1989) 'The housing question', in Herbert, D.T. and Smith, D.M. (eds) *Social Problems and the City* (Oxford: Oxford University Press)

Kerr, M. and Charles, N. (1983) *Attitudes to the Feeding and Nutrition of Young Children*: *Preliminary report* (York: University of York)

Kiernan, K. (1989) 'The family: formation and fission', in Joshi, H. (ed.) *The Changing Population of Britain* (Oxford: Blackwell)

Kiernan, K. and Wicks, M. (1990) *Family Change and Future Policy* (London: Family Policy Studies Centre)

Kleinman, M. and Whitehead, C.M.E. (1988) 'The prospects for private renting in the 1990s', in Kemp, P. (ed.) *The Private Provision of Rented Housing* (Aldershot: Gower)

Land, H. (1992) 'Families and the law', in Cochrane, A. and Muncie, J. (eds) *Politics, Policy and the Law* (Milton Keynes: Open University)

Lee, P. and Gibney, M. (1989) *Patterns of Food and Nutrient Intake in a Suburb of Dublin with Chronically High Unemployment* (Dublin: Combat Poverty Agency)

Leira, A. (1987) 'Time for work, time for care: childcare strategies in a Norwegian setting', in Brannen, J. and Wilson, G. (eds) *Give and Take in Families*: *Studies in resource distribution* (London: Allen & Unwin)

Levy, E.F. (1989) 'Lesbian motherhood: identity and social support' *Affilia*, vol.4, no.4, pp.40–53

Lewis, J. and Bowlby, S. (1989) 'Women's inequality in urban Britain', in Herbert, D.T. and Smith, D.M. (eds) *Social Problems and the City* (Oxford: Oxford University Press)

Lewis, J. and Meredith, B. (1988) *Daughters Who Care*: *Daughters caring for mothers at home* (London: Routledge)

Lister, R. (1991) 'Overhaul of maintenance', *Poverty*, vol.78, pp.11–13

Littlewood, J. and Tinker, A. (1981) *Families in Flats* (London: Department of Environment, HMSO)

Lonsdale, S. (1990) *Women and Disability: The experience of physical disability among women* (London: Macmillan)

Lyman, P. (1981) 'The politics of anger: on silence, resentment and political speech', *Socialist Review*, vol.3, pp.55–74

MacPike, L. (ed.) (1989) *There's Something I've Been Meaning to Tell You* (Tallahassee, USA: Naiad Press)

McEwen, C. and O'Sullivan, S. (eds) (1988) *Out the Other Side: Contemporary lesbian writing* (London: Virago Press)

McKeith, C. (1992) 'Maresa' in Morris, J. (ed.) *Alone Together: Voices of single mothers* (London: Women's Press)

McRae, S. and Daniel, W.W. (1991) *Maternity Rights: The experience of women and employers* (London: Policy Studies Institute)

Mama, A. (1989) *The Hidden Struggle: Statutory and voluntary sector responses to violence against black women in the home* (London: London Race and Housing Research Unit)

Mansfield, B. (1989) 'The mother from outer space' in L. MacPike (ed.) *There's Something I've Been Meaning to Tell You* (Tallahassee, USA: Naiad Press)

Martin, J., Meltzer, H. and Elliot, D. (1988) *The Prevalence of Disability Among Adults* (London: OPCS Surveys of Disability in Great Britain, Report 1, HMSO)

Martin, J. and Roberts, C. (1984) *Women and Employment* (London: Department of Employment and OPCS Report, HMSO)

Martin, J. and White, A. (1988) *The Financial Circumstances of Disabled Adults Living in Private Households* (London: OPCS Surveys of Disability in Great Britain, Report 2, HMSO)

Martin, J., White, A. and Meltzer, H. (1989) *Disabled Adults: Services, transport and employment* (London: OPCS Surveys of Disability in Great Britain, Report 4, HMSO)

Mason, M. (1991) 'Able parents – disability, pregnancy and motherhood', *Maternity Action*, vol.51, pp.9–10

Mason, M. (1992) 'A nineteen-parent family' in Morris, J. (ed.) *Alone Together: Voices of single mothers* (London: Women's Press)

Maternity Action (1992a) 'Frozen Thrice', *Maternity Action*, vol.53, p.11

Maternity Action (1992b) 'Young pregnant women', *Maternity Action*, vol.53, pp.8–9

Mayall, B. (1986) *Keeping Children Healthy* (London: Allen & Unwin)

Meltzer, H., Smyth, M. and Robus, N. (1989) *Disabled Children: Services, transport and education*, (London: OPCS Surveys of Disability in Great Britain, Report 6, HMSO)

Millar, J. (1989) *Poverty and the Lone-parent Family: The challenge to social policy* (Aldershot, Hants: Avebury)

Millar, J. (1991) 'Bearing the cost' in Becker, S. (ed.) *Windows of Opportunity: Public policy and the poor* (London: Child Poverty Action Group)

Miller, M. (1990) *Bed and Breakfast: Women and homelessness today* (London: Women's Press)

Morris, J. (1989) *Able Lives: Women's experience of paralysis* (London: Women's Press)

Morris, J. (1990) *Our Homes, Our Rights: Housing, independent living and physically disabled people* (London: Shelter)

Morris, J. (1991) *Pride Against Prejudice: Transforming attitudes to disability* (London: Women's Press)

Morris, J. (ed.) (1992a) *Alone Together: Voices of single mothers* (London: Women's Press)

Morris, J. (1992b) 'Feeling special', in Morris, J. (ed.) *Alone Together: Voices of single mothers* (London: Women's Press)

Morris, L. (1983) 'Redundancy and patterns of household finance', *Sociological Review*, vol.32, no.3, pp.492–523

Morris, L. (1987) 'Constraints on gender: the family wage, social security and the labour market', *Work, Employment and Society*, vol.1, no.1, pp.85–106

Morris, L. (1990) *The Workings of the Household* (Cambridge: Polity Press)

Morris, L. (1991) 'Women's poor work', in Brown, P. and Scase, R. (eds) *Poor Work: Disadvantage and the division of labour* (Milton Keynes: Open University Press)

Morrow, V. (1992) *Family Values: Accounting for children's contribution to the domestic economy* (Cambridge: Working Paper No.10, Sociological Research Group)

Morton, C. (1991) 'Family law – recent changes', *Rights of Women Bulletin*, Winter 1990/1, pp.7–11

Moss, P. (1991) 'Day care for young children in the United Kingdom', in Melhuish, E.C. and Moss, P. (eds) *Day Care for Young Children: International perspectives* (London: Routledge)

Murray, P. (1992) 'Jessie and Kim' in Morris, J. (ed.) *Alone Together: Voices of single mothers* (London: Women's Press)

National Association of Citizens Advice Bureaux (1991) *Barriers to Benefit: Black claimants and social security* (London: National Association of Citizens Advice Bureaux)

New Review (1991a) 'The rise and rise of low pay', *The New Review*, vol.7, pp.11–14

New Review (1991b) 'Part-time work: double bad deal', *The New Review*, vol.8, pp.12–15

Oakley, A. (1979) *Becoming a Mother* (Oxford: Martin Robertson)

Office of Population Censuses and Surveys (1988) *Occupational Mortality, Childhood Supplement, 1979–80, 1982–3*, Series DS No.8 (London: HMSO)

Office of Population Censuses and Surveys (1990a) *General Household Survey 1988* (London: HMSO)

Office of Population Censuses and Surveys (1990b) *Morbidity Statistics from General Practice, 1981–82; Socio-economic analysis*, Series MB5(1) (London: HMSO)

Office of Population Censuses and Surveys (1991a) *General Household Survey 1989* (London: HMSO)

Office of Population Censuses and Surveys (1991b) *Labour Force Survey 1988 and 1989*, Series LFS No.8 (London: HMSO)

Office of Population Censuses and Surveys (1991c) *Mortality Statistics, Perinatal and Infant: Social and biological factors*, Series DH3, No.22 (London: HMSO)

Office of Population Censuses and Surveys (1991d) *General Household Survey: Cigarette smoking 1972–1990*, SS91/3 (London: OPCS)

Office of Population Censuses and Surveys (1991e) *Mortality Statistics, Childhood, England and Wales*, Series DH6, No.3 (London: HMSO)

Office of Population Censuses and Surveys (1992) *Mortality Statistics, Perinatal and Infant: Social and biological factors*, Series DH3 No.23 (London: HMSO)

O'Higgins, M. (1989) 'Inequality, social policy and income distribution in the United Kingdom', in Jallode, J.-P. (ed.) *The Crisis of Redistribution in European Welfare States* (Stoke: Trentham Books)

Ohri, S. (1988) 'The politics of racism, statistics and equal opportunity: towards a black perspective', in Bhat, A., Carr-Hill, R. and Ohri, S. (eds) *Britain's Black Population* (Aldershot: Gower)

Oliver, M. (1990) *The Politics of Disablement* (London: Macmillan)

Oppenheim, C. (1990) *Poverty: The facts* (London: Child Poverty Action Group)

O'Sullivan, S. and Thomson, K. (eds) (1992) *Positively Women: Living with AIDS* (London: Sheba)

Pahl, J. (1985) 'Marital violence and marital breakdown', in Pahl, J. (ed.) *Private Violence and Public Policy* (London: Routledge & Kegan Paul)

Pahl, J. (1989) *Money and Marriage* (London: Macmillan)

Pahl, R.E. (1984) *Divisions of Labour* (Oxford: Blackwell)

Payne, S. (1991) *Women, Health and Poverty* (Hemel Hempstead: Harvester Wheatsheaf)

Pearson, M., Dawson, C., Spencer, S. and Moore, H. (1992) *Inter-household Dependency: The poor relation in health care behaviour* (Liverpool: Working Paper No.4, Department of Economics and Accounting, University of Liverpool)

Phillips, E. (1992) 'Bringing up Ella', in Morris, J. (ed.) *Alone Together: Voices of single mothers* (London: Women's Press)

Phizacklea, A. (1982) 'Migrant women and wage labour: the case of West Indian women in Britain', in West, J. (ed.) *Work, Women and the Labour Market* (London: Routledge & Kegan Paul)

Phizacklea, A. (1988) 'Entrepreneurship, ethnicity and gender', in Westwood, S. and Bhachu, P. (eds) *Enterprising Women: Ethnicity, economy and gender relations* (London: Routledge)

Phoenix, A. (1988) 'Narrow definitions of culture', in Westwood, S. and Bhachu, P. (eds) *Enterprising Women: Ethnicity, economy and gender relations* (London: Routledge)

Phoenix, A. (1991) *Young Mothers?* (London: Polity Press)

Phoenix, A., Woollett, A. and Lloyd, E. (eds) (1991) *Motherhood: Meanings, practices and ideologies* (London: Sage)

Piachaud, D. (1984) *Round About 50 Hours a Week: The time costs of children* (London: Child Poverty Action Group)

Piachaud, D. (1986) *Poor Children: A tale of two decades* (London: Child Poverty Action Group)

Pill, R. and Stott, N. (1982) 'Concepts of illness causation and responsibility: some preliminary data from a sample of working class mothers', *Social Science and Medicine*, vol.16, pp.43–52

Platt, S.D., Martin, C.J., Hunt, S.M. and Lewis, C.W. (1989) 'Damp housing, mould growth and symptomatic health state', *British Medical Journal*, vol.298, pp.1673–8

Plummer, K. (1983) *Documents of Life* (London: Allen and Unwin)

Pollert, A. (1981) *Girls, Wives and Factory Lives* (London: Macmillan)

Popay, J. (1989) 'Poverty and plenty: women's experiences across social classes', in Graham, H. and Popay, J. (eds) *Women and Poverty: Exploring the research and policy agenda* (London: Thomas Coram Research Unit/University of Warwick)

Popay, J. (1992) ' "My health is all right, but I'm just tired all the time": women's experiences of ill-health', in Roberts, H. (ed.) *Women's Health Matters* (London: Routledge)

Popay, J. and Bartley, M. (1989) 'Conditions of labour and women's health', in Martin, C. and McQueen, D. (eds) *Readings in the New Public Health* (Edinburgh: Edinburgh University Press)

Popay, J. and Jones, G. (1990) 'Patterns of health and illness amongst lone parents', *Journal of Social Policy*, vol.19, no.4, pp.499–534

Pugh, H., Power, C., Goldblatt, P. and Arber, S. (1991) 'Women's lung cancer mortality, socio-economic status and changing smoking patterns', *Social Science and Medicine*, vol.32, no.10, pp.1105–10

Quick, A. (1991) *Unequal Risks* (London: Socialist Health Association)

Rao, N. (1990) *Black Women in Public Sector Housing* (London: Commission for Racial Equality)

Raynsford, N. (1989) 'Housing', in McCarthy, M. (ed.) *The New Politics of Welfare* (London: Macmillan)

Read, J. (1991) 'There was never really any choice: the experience of mothers of disabled children in the United Kingdom', *Women's Studies International Forum*, vol.14, no.6, pp.561–71

Richman, N., Stevenson, J. and Graham, P. (1982) *Preschool to School: A behavioural study* (London: Academic Press)

Rights of Women Lesbian Custody Group (1986) *Lesbian Mothers' Legal Handbook* (London: Women's Press)

Ritchie, J. (1990) *Thirty Families: Their living standards in unemployment* (London: HMSO)

Robinson, V. (1989) 'Economic restructuring, the urban crisis and Britain's black population', in Herbert, D.T. and Smith, D.M. (eds) *Social Problems and the City* (Oxford: Oxford University Press)

Rodrigues, L. and Botting, B. (1989) 'Recent trends in postneonatal mortality in England', *Population Trends*, vol.55, pp.7–15

Roll, J. (1991) *What Is a Family?: Benefit models and social realities* (London: Family Policy Studies Centre)

Rose, E.J.B. (1969) *Colour and Citizenship: A report on British race relations* (London: Oxford University Press)

Ross, M. (1988) 'Pushing the boundaries', in Grewal, S., Kay, J., Landor, L., Lewis, G. and Parmar, P. (eds) *Charting the Journey: Writings by black and third world women* (London: Sheba Feminist Publishers)

Sadiq, A. (1991) 'Asian women and the benefit system', *FSU Quarterly*, vol.46, pp.42–7

Sadiq-Sangster, A. (1991) *Just About Surviving: life on income support: An Asian experience* (London: Family Service Units)

Salvat, G. (1989) 'Gilli Salvat', in Hall Carpenter Archives/Lesbian Oral History Group (ed.) *Inventing Ourselves: Lesbian Life Stories* (London: Routledge)

Scott, J. (1990) *A Matter of Record: Documentary sources in social research* (London: Polity Press)

Sexty, C. (1990) *Women Losing Out: Access to housing in Britain today* (London: Shelter)

Sharpe, S. (1984) *Double Identity: The lives of working mothers* (Harmondsworth: Penguin)

Shaw, M. and Miles, I. (1979) 'The social roots of statistical knowledge', in Irvine, J., Miles, I. and Evans, J. (eds) *Demystifying Social Statistics* (London: Pluto Press)

Simms, M. and Smith, C. (1986) *Teenage Mothers and their Partners* (London: Research Report No.15, HMSO)

Skellington, R. (1993) 'Homelessness', in Dallos, R. and McLaughlin, E. (eds) *Social Problems and the Family* (London: Sage)

Smyth, M. and Robus, N. (1989) *The Financial Circumstances of Families with Disabled Children Living in Private Households* (London: OPCS Surveys of Disability in Great Britain, Report 5, HMSO)

Snitow, A. (1992) 'Feminism and motherhood: an American reading', *Feminist Review*, vol.40, pp.32–51

Solomos, J. (1989) *Race and Racism in Contemporary Britain* (London: Macmillan)

Steedman, C. (1986) *Landscape for a Good Woman* (London: Virago Press)

Stone, K. (1983) 'Motherhood and waged work: West Indian, Asian and white mothers compared', in Phizacklea, A. (ed.) *One Way Ticket: Migration and female labour* (London: Routledge & Kegan Paul)

Strachan, D.P. (1988) 'Damp housing and childhood asthma: validation of reporting symptoms', *British Medical Journal*, vol.297, pp.1223–6

Taking Liberties Collective (1989) *Learning the Hard Way: Women's oppression in men's education* (London: Macmillan)

Thomas, A. and Niner, P. (1989) *Living in Temporary Accommodation: A study of homeless people* (London: HMSO)

Thornton, R. (1990) *The New Homeless* (London: Housing Centre Bookshop)

Ungerson, C. (1987) *Policy is Personal: Sex, gender and informal care* (London: Tavistock)

Verbrugge, L.M. (1985) 'Gender and health: an update on hypotheses and evidence', *Journal of Health and Social Behaviour*, vol.26, pp.156–62

Wadsworth, M.E.J. (1991) *The Imprint of Time: Childhood, history and adult life* (Oxford: Clarendon Press)

Walker, B. (1992) 'A woman's right to choose', in Morris, J. (ed.) *Alone Together: Voices of single mothers* (London: Women's Press)

Walsh, A. and Lister, R. (1985) *Mother's Life-line: A survey of how women use and value child benefit* (London: Child Poverty Action Group)

Warrier, S. (1988) 'Marriage, maternity and female economic activity', in Westwood, S. and Bhachu, P. (eds) *Enterprising Women: Ethnicity, economy and gender relations* (London: Routledge)

Wates, M. (1991) 'Able parents – disability, pregnancy and motherhood', *Maternity Action*, vol.52, pp.9–10

Wells, J. (1987) *Women and Smoking: An evaluation of the role of stress in smoking cessation and relapse* (Southampton: Department of Psychology, University of Southampton)

Wells, N. (1987) *Women's Health Today* (London: Office of Health Economics)

White, P. (1990) 'A question on ethnic group for the census: findings from the 1989 census test post-enumeration survey', *Population Trends*, vol.59, pp.11–20

Williams, C. (1988) 'Gal . . . you come from foreign', in Grewal, S., Kay, J., Landor, L., Lewis, G. and Parmar, P. (eds) *Charting the Journey: Writings by black and third world women* (London: Sheba Feminist Publishers)

Wilmott, P. (1987) *Friendship Networks and Social Support* (London: Policy Studies Institute)

Wilson, A. (1978) *Finding a Voice: Asian women in Britain* (London: Virago Press)

Witherspoon, S. (1988) 'Interim report: a woman's work', in Jowell, R., Witherspoon, S. and Brook, L. (eds) *British Social Attitudes: The 5th report* (Aldershot: Gower)

Witherspoon, S. and Prior, S. (1991) 'Working mothers: free to choose?', in Jowell, R., Brook, L. and Taylor, B. (eds) *British Social Attitudes: The 8th report* (Aldershot: Dartmouth Publishing Co.)

Woollett, A. (1991) 'Having children: accounts of childless women and women with reproductive problems', in Phoenix, A., Woollett, A. and Lloyd, E. (eds) *Motherhood: Meanings, practices and ideologies* (London: Sage)

INDEX